The Emotionally Intelligent Social Worker

Also by David Howe:

Social Workers and their Practices in Welfare Bureaucracies
An Introduction to Social Work Theory
The Consumers' View of Family Therapy
Half a Million Women: Mothers who Lose their Children by Adoption
 (with Phillida Sawbridge and Diana Hinings)
*Attachment Theory for Social Workers**
Attachment and Loss in Child and Family Social Work
Adopters on Adoption: Reflections on Parenthood and Childhood
Patterns of Adoption: Nature, Nurture and Psychosocial Development
*Attachment Theory, Child Maltreatment and Family Support**
 (with M. Brandon, D. Hinings and G. Schofield)
Adoption, Search and Reunion (with J. Feast)
The Adoption Reunion Handbook (with L. Trinder and J. Feast)
Contact in Adoption and Permanent Foster Care (with E. Neil)
*Child Abuse and Neglect: Attachment, Development and Intervention**

* *also published by Palgrave Macmillan*

The Emotionally Intelligent Social Worker

David Howe

palgrave
macmillan

KH

First published 2008 by
PALGRAVE MACMILLAN
Houndmills, Basingstoke, Hampshire RG21 6XS and
175 Fifth Avenue, New York, N.Y. 10010
Companies and representatives throughout the world

PALGRAVE MACMILLAN is the global academic imprint of the Palgrave Macmillan division of St. Martin's Press, LLC and of Palgrave Macmillan Ltd. Macmillan® is a registered trademark in the United States, United Kingdom and other countries. Palgrave is a registered trademark in the European Union and other countries.

ISBN-13: 978–0–230–20278–8
ISBN-10: 0–230–20278–0

This book is printed on paper suitable for recycling and made from fully managed and sustained forest sources. Logging, pulping and manufacturing processes are expected to conform to the environmental regulations of the country of origin.

A catalogue record for this book is available from the British Library.

A catalog record for this book is available from the Library of Congress.

10   9   8   7   6   5   4   3   2   1
17   16   15   14   13   12   11   10   09   08

Printed and bound in China

9/3/09

For Jacob, Angela, Rebecca, Matt . . . and Elsa.

Acknowledgements

I should like to thank Catherine Gray of Palgrave Macmillan for her patience, support and encouragement over the last thirteen years. Catherine's astute observations and advice have always been helpful. I am also grateful for the perceptive comments of two anonymous reviewers. Their thoughts have been happily taken into account. Naturally, I remain responsible for the final version of the present book, including its imperfections, inelegancies, and any mistakes it may contain.

David Howe
Norwich

Contents

1
Once More With Feeling

Introduction

We are creatures saturated by feelings. We are a species that can love and hate. Having a strong sense of past, present and future, we can worry about what we have done, what we might do, and what might happen. It is because we are social beings that we are also emotional beings. Many of our strongest feelings arise in relationship with others: envy and shame, desire and regret, sadness and joy. In this book, I want to argue that the more we understand ourselves at the level of feeling, the wiser we become. Certainly, being intelligent about emotions and the part they play in our lives makes us socially more skilled. Knowing when to contain anger, knowing when to say nothing rather than something, understanding the value of a kind word at the right time, recognizing the need to stay with someone who is hurt rather than dismiss them as out-of-control, these are examples of emotional intelligence. It is this kind of intelligence that marks out personal success and wellbeing.

The people-oriented professions inevitably find themselves working daily with people whose needs are pressing and whose emotions are disturbingly aroused. Illness, physical decline, and poverty increase anxiety. Injustice, deprivation and discrimination provoke anger. Loss and rejection leave people feeling hurt and sad. It is critical that social and health care workers understand the fundamental part that emotions play in the lives and behaviour of those who use their services. Emotions define the character of the professional relationship. Practitioners need to understand how emotions affect them as they work with users and engage with colleagues.

This, then, is a book about the emotions – what they are, why we have them, how they affect us, how they colour relationships. Social and health care work is emotional work of a high order whether it's with older people, children and families, offenders, disabled children and adults, or the mentally ill. The more intelligent practitioners are

1

about emotions and the part they play in health and health care work, the more sensitive, thoughtful and effective will be their practice. Emotional intelligence is therefore a core skill without which practice would not only be ineffective, it would lack humanity.

Reason and Emotion

The term *emotional intelligence* has captured the popular imagination. Although there were precursors, emotional intelligence was first discussed in earnest in the early 1990s when its use spread quickly in the media and popular science. People who were emotionally literate appeared to do well at school and were successful at work. They were good at social relationships. Indeed, it was not long before some argued that emotional intelligence should rank alongside, or even above cognitive intelligence in importance. And individuals fortunate to be in possession of both types of intelligence were said to be doubly blessed. It was highly likely that life would give them an easy ride.

Psychology has always suspected that success and competence are not governed by one general type of intelligence. There are horses for courses; those who are good at one activity are likely to have one kind of 'intelligence', while those skilled at another will be supported by a different innate talent. A gifted dancer, a brilliant footballer, or an imaginative artist might be at least as successful in life as the more conventional academically 'intelligent' individual. Sternberg (1985) was impressed by people who had what he called *practical intelligence*. Individuals in possession of this intelligence, knowing what to do in a given situation, got on and did it whether or not it involved the use of intellectual, physical or social wit. Gardner (1983, 1993) talked of 'multiple intelligences'. He identified 'intelligences' that were linguistic, spatial, logical-mathematical, musical, bodily-kinaesthetic ('athletic'), *intra*personal, and *inter*personal. Emotional intelligence is roughly defined by these last two, and it is these two that social workers need in good measure.

There is evidence that there is considerable overlap between many of these intelligences, particularly those involving the use of practical, social and emotional skills. This trio appears to work particularly well in situations which do not lend themselves to straightforward, correct, single answer solutions. However, in broad terms we might recognize two kinds of mind: one that thinks and one that feels.

Goleman (1995: 8) wonders whether interactions between these two fundamentally different ways of knowing might in fact 'construct our mental life'. We shall be paying particular attention to the mind that feels.

Of course, there is a problem writing about the emotions. Writing requires thought and thoughts have to be organized, ideas ordered. Books are a product of the mind, of cognition. They demand structure. But the emotions speak of a different world. They colour experience. A feeling can agitate the body every bit as much it can trouble the mind. A mood can cloud a day or excite a week. We challenge those whose emotions are running high to show calm and be reasonable. We accuse those who are all head and no heart of being cold and unfeeling.

For the first half of the 20th century, psychologists got round the problem of writing about the emotions by dismissing their importance, at least as far as the scientific study of human behaviour was concerned. They either ignored feelings or saw them as a contaminant to the proper study of people and their behaviour. Although several pioneering 19th century scientists, including Charles Darwin, Sigmund Freud, and William James, saw emotions as central to the task of enquiring about human psychology, by the 1920s behaviourists were dismissing the emotions as worthy of scientific study. The later 'cognitive revolution' in the 1950s also had little time for the emotions. But lest we be too harsh, these early behavioural and cognitive psychologists were merely the latest in a long line of thinkers who remained suspicious of the part that the emotions might play in understanding the human mind.

Forgas (2001a) writes that 'Many philosophers, starting with Plato, have traditionally assumed that affect has a dangerous, invasive quality on rational thinking and behaviour' (p xv). The Stoics of ancient Greece also believed that feelings undermined rational thought. If we are to lead the good life, they argued, we should not allow ourselves to be at the mercy of our passions. If our actions are to be rational, we should overcome our base emotions using the power of reason and logic. Centuries later, many Western philosophers including St Augustine, Descartes, and Kant continued to see the emotions as basic, primitive, disruptive. Human enlightenment, they believed, required that we rid ourselves of animal passion and rise above emotion.

But those of a more artistic temperament have always rejected the rationalist's distrust of feeling. A number of Enlightenment philosophers, including David Hume and Adam Smith, understood that, along with reason, the emotions were an integral part of our individual and collective psychology. Only when reason and emotion are working in harmony is intelligent action possible. Others went beyond even this arguing that emotions are fundamentally at odds with reason (Evans 2001: xii). Flourishing in the 18th century, the European Romantic movement rode the waves of untamed passion and positively embraced the life-enhancing power of the emotions. Truth and authenticity are to be found in the contemplation of nature. Emotion and human passion lie deep in the heart of the natural world. In contrast to the Rationalists, Rousseau believed that reason was the problem not passion. To recover our wellbeing, he felt, we have to return to an innocent state of nature.

In the hands of the Romantics, art becomes the expression of emotion (Collingwood 1938). Painters and poets celebrated intuition and mocked logic, revelled in empathy and eschewed science. They preferred the pastoral, fleeing the city as the tentacles of urban life spread the ugly grip of science and industry ever wider. It is art's business to explore, value and express the natural world, a world which includes human minds and relationships, whether in prose or poetry, painting or music. Our relationship with the world of things and people is a thoroughly emotional one and it is the role of art to examine this. 'If a story doesn't work emotionally', wrote Martel, 'it does not work at all' (1993: p viii cited in Cozolino 2006: 66). Robinson (2007) agrees. In her examination of the role that emotions play in literature, music and art, she suggests that great writing, symphonies and painting have to be experienced emotionally if they are properly to be understood. Gérard, a character in Forster's novel about the artist Gwen John, says 'Paintings are feelings. It doesn't matter what the eye sees, the heart must feel, or it is useless' (Forster 2007: 328). Reason and critical thought on their own are dry and without passion. It is only when art engages us emotionally that connections are made, experience expands, and understanding, not just of the novel or poem, piano piece or picture, but also of ourselves, deepens.

It is also the case that we seek out artistic experiences in order to excite and intensify our emotions. The pursuit of pleasure makes us happy, even ecstatic. However, we can also appreciate artistic experiences that cause us sorrow (a play based on a tragedy), or make us angry (a politically inspired painting or photograph), frightened (a horror film), or sad (a moving piece of music). There is a sense of being alive whenever our passions are roused and heightened. These aesthetic experiences help us to feel, explore and think about many of the common conditions that affect humanity and in so doing they raise our understanding and sympathies. The arts and humanities, being explorations of the meaning of experience, can therefore help us develop our emotional intelligence and make us more compassionate and decent beings.

Being Acknowledged

Although disdain of the emotions might have been true of some mid-twentieth century academic psychologists, many of those at the applied end of the discipline knew better. Their daily experience was one in which the passions were all too often careering out-of-control, de-railing relationships, creating problems at work, making people feel unhappy and even unwell. Folk wisdom has always understood that the heart as much as the head is the source of feeling, that the body as well as the mind is involved in emotion. 'The heart', wrote Blasé Pascal (1643/1966: 113), 'has its reasons which reason knows nothing of'.

We also capture something of the insights generated by folk psychology when we ask those who have been on the receiving end of social work, counselling and psychotherapy to evaluate the experience. Client views and the perspective of service users have a habit of talking about the technical business of providing a professional service in a direct, down-to-earth, feeling-based way. 'The nearer we stay to common speech', believes Lomas (1981), 'the less likely we are to destroy the meaning of those who seek our help'. Clients and service users value the quality of the relationship and the things that promote it including how they feel about the social worker and how the social worker makes them feel. For example, users positively rate social workers who they see as 'warm and friendly' (Strupp 1969: 17). They value help which feels supportive.

Maluccio (1979: 61) discovered that when counsellors are asked to recall the first session, they mention the problems presented. However, when clients are asked the same question, they remember their feelings, including how the counsellor made them feel. It seems that when our emotions run high, most of us tend to talk more. Talk also turns out to be part of the medium in which the self forms and re-forms in which we try to mend our broken and hurt selves (Howe 1993). So, the emotional tone of the worker-user relationship is critical to therapeutic success.

One of the hallmarks of a good relationship is that our feelings, however dark and distressing, are recognized, understood and accepted by the other. If the relationship is a place where we can feel safe, then we can explore the thoughts and feelings that are distorting and disfiguring our lives. A daughter might admit: 'I know I shouldn't feel so angry with my ageing mother, but her growing dependence and forgetfulness irritate me and I'm surprised and alarmed at the aggression I feel.' Or the stressed father of an autistic son confesses: 'My longed for son seems no more interested in me than his toy cars. I suppose I am disappointed. I'm not sure I like him. How can I possibly be feeling this way? I feel wretched.' For service users, such feelings are real, but hard to face up to. It is up to the social worker and the care worker to offer a relationship where it feels safe to recognize and explore the emotions that trouble and cause pain.

Talking of her own experiences of being in psychotherapy, France (1988: 111) believes that 'what is needed is a friendly therapist, the creation of space where you are entitled to be just who you are, however defective'. Only then can you feel understood, only then can the serious business of addressing the hurt and the harm begin. It is vital that the social worker and the counsellor, the therapist and the care worker create a space where it is safe for the service user to admit feelings and to let down anxiously held-on to defences.

> The more I felt secure in the feeling of being accepted as me, not necessarily liked, but responded to as an individual, the more I felt I was able to explore this self, and its more unsavoury aspects. (France 1988: 242)

Empathy, acceptance and not judging the other allows people to acknowledge and accept what they think and feel. They don't have to run and hide, defend and deny. There is someone prepared to stay with them. The simple presence of another who is strong enough to 'hold' the relationship and the user's difficult emotions in itself can be therapeutic. Service users no longer feel demeaned by their base emotions, they do not feel diminished. As feelings are described, the social practitioner is also giving the message that the individual is worth listening to and worth understanding.

So it is that a knowledge and understanding of our own and other people's emotions is key to the helping process. The social worker who is emotionally intelligent is more than half way to being an effective social worker.

Understanding Feelings and Feeling Understood

It has been rather late in the day that the psychological research community has begun to catch up with what everyone else knew: that not only are the emotions of great importance in the conduct of everyday life, but they also define what makes us human. 'Should we not define ourselves as those beings that can love and make commitments, that suffer grief at losing someone irreplaceable, and that feel shame at having behaved badly?' (Oatley 1998: 285). This is why the computer brain will never be like the human brain, no matter how much information it processes or rational logic it acquires. To be human, computers would need to experience the world at the level of feeling. 'If computers want to think', declares Hobson (2002: xv), 'they had better get a social life'. Tomkins (1962: 112) felt that 'reason without affect would be impotent, affect without reason would be blind'. Emotions may, in fact, be vital to intelligent action (Evans and Cruse 2004).

Better late than never, the last twenty years has seen an explosion of research and writing on the emotions. It is this more recent work that will inform much of this book. Not surprisingly, given the fundamental and universal character of the emotions, many of the psychosocial sciences as well as the humanities have much to say on matters of feeling. If we are to do justice to the subject, we shall need to engage the thoughts of psychologists and psychiatrists, biologists and neuroscientists, philosophers and anthropologists.

In the following pages, we define emotional intelligence (Chapter Two). Evolutionary theory forms a backcloth to these early discussions. How we cope with stress – or not – also plays a part in our understanding. Feelings have an elusive quality. Quite what they are or why we have them is not immediately obvious. We all know what it is like to feel happy or sad, but what are these subjective states? What exactly are emotions? These questions need attention (Chapter Three).

The development of the emotions from infancy to adulthood also takes us on a wonderful journey, particularly as it tells us something about the social nature of our selves and what it is to be human (Chapter Four). At this point in the story we shall meet the brain scientists (Chapter Five). They have many interesting things to say about the emotions and the ways in which we learn to understand and regulate them, particularly in the context of close relationships. Closely tied to these issues is the relationship between stress, coping and our physical health (Chapter Six). Emotional wellbeing affects not only our mental health but also our physical health. The growth of 'positive psychology' or the science of happiness is a reminder that the mind and the body are intimately connected. Unfortunately, for some children their journey across the seas of emotional development is anything but smooth. The quality of their care is poor, social relationships are difficult. This takes us into the troubled waters of emotional disorders, behavioural difficulties and relationship problems both in children and adults (Chapter Seven).

Helping service users and clients to feel in control of their lives, to be able to regulate their emotions, and to achieve emotional wellbeing is what much of social work is about. There is a strong case to be made that helping people manage their emotions and cope with stress is the basis of most interventions and therapies. We shall consider social work help, support and treatment in terms of recognizing, understanding and learning to manage distress and emotional arousal (Chapters Eight and Nine).

Conclusion

The emotionally intelligent social worker understands the part that emotions play in her own and other people's thoughts and feelings, hopes and beliefs, designs and plans, behaviour and perceptions. She can use this knowledge with skill and sensitivity to engage with those in distress and difficulty. She is intelligent about what emotions are, about how they affect us. The emotionally intelligent worker knows what emotions are and how they can be managed, developed and used in the self and others. The social work profession, particularly during its early development, has always understood that emotions lie at the heart of its concerns. Let us now examine the emergence and growth of 'emotional intelligence' – as a concept, a skill, indeed as a defining feature of the socially gifted.

2
What is Emotional Intelligence?

Introduction

The argument that emotional intelligence is of fundamental important across most domains of human functioning has, perhaps, been
overstated. Even so, it might be reasonable to argue that the professions that work with people, particularly people in need and distress,
should be populated by individuals in goodly possession of
emotional intelligence. Social work is one such profession. It deals
with people who are troubled and troubling. It enters the frame when
emotions are running high. Social workers find themselves trying to
help the frightened victims of domestic violence; older people who
sink into depression as their mobility declines and independence
ebbs away; disabled people who feel mounting anger as they try to
move around in a world of steps and narrow doorways so thought-
lessly designed by and for those who can walk and squeeze and
climb. If social workers are to understand and manage their own and
other people's feelings in these emotionally charged situations, then
social workers will need to be emotionally intelligent.

Conceptual Beginnings

A precursor of emotional intelligence was the concept of social intelligence. Thorndike (1920) defined socially intelligent people as individuals who possess keen psychological insight, social sensitivity,
empathy and social adaptability. They are active rather than passive
participants in their own lives (Zirkel 2000: 3). They respond well to
new situations. All of this makes them good communicators, skilful
group members, and social problem-solvers.

As early as 1960, Mowrer concluded that the emotions 'do not at all
deserve being put in opposition with "intelligence" . . . they are, it
seems, a high order of intelligence' (pp 307–8). This suggests that
emotions play a key part in the way we perceive, understand and

reason about people and things. Around this time the idea that there was such a thing as emotional intelligence was beginning to crop up in variety of different fields including literary criticism and psychiatry (Mayer et al 2004: 198). Credit for first coining the actual term 'emotional intelligence' in psychology is often given to Wayne Leon Payne. In 1985 he published his doctoral thesis titled *A Study of Emotion: Developing Emotional Intelligence.* Payne believed that the civilized world's tendency to suppress emotion stifles the growth of emotional intelligence. This leads to emotional ignorance and a variety of mental health problems including depression, aggression, and addiction.

A few years later in a seminal paper with the title 'Emotional Intelligence', Salovey and Mayer (1990) conceptually clarified the idea that people who understand the part that the emotions play in their own and other people's psychological lives also seem to be socially very skilled. Their paper set in motion a great bandwagon of research and writing on the subject of emotional intelligence.

However, it was the journalist and psychologist Daniel Goleman who argued that emotional intelligence was every bit as important to success in life as cognitive intelligence. His book, *Emotional Intelligence,* first published in 1995, became an international best seller. There was something about the idea of using and understanding emotions intelligently that seemed to hit the spot. The term quickly became fashionable amongst management consultants, trainers, education-alists, mental health specialists, and those in the media. In its first blush, the benefits claimed for being emotionally intelligent were often extravagant. Emotionally intelligent children were said to be the most academically successful. Emotionally literate managers would boost the productivity of their workforce. Popularity would be the reward of the emotionally savvy politician. There is some truth in these claims but more recent research and reflection has tempered some of the wilder assertions. We are now in possession of a more measured understanding of the undoubted importance of emotional intelligence in human affairs.

Definitions

At the heart of emotional intelligence is the ability to understand both our selves and other people as emotional beings. The emotion-ally intelligent person understands that emotions affect behaviour, beliefs, perceptions, interpretations, thoughts and actions. The ability to adjust, modify and regulate our emotions as we relate with others is also a key element of emotional intelligence. Fischer et al (2004) feel that 'individuals who do not respond emotionally in an adequate manner may survive physically, but will become social outcasts' (p 188). Gardner saw two linked aspects of emotional intelligence – the interpersonal and the intrapersonal:

> *Inter*personal intelligence is the ability to understand other people: what motivates them, how they work, how to work cooperatively with them. Successful salespeople, politicians, teachers, clinicians, and religious leaders are all likely to be individuals with high degrees of interpersonal intelligence. *Intra*personal intelligence . . . is a correlative ability, turned inward. It is a capacity to form an accurate, veridical model of oneself and to be able to use that model to operate effectively in life. (Gardner 1993: 9)

Salovey and Mayer (1990) raised the concept of emotional intelligence one further level. In 2004, Mayer et al offered a general working definition of emotional intelligence as:

> the capacity to reason about emotions, and of emotions to enhance thinking. It includes the abilities to accurately perceive emotions, to access and generate emotions so as to assist thought, to understand emotions and emotional knowledge, and to reflectively regulate emotions so as to promote emotional and intellectual growth. (Mayer et al 2004: 197)

They see emotional intelligence as just one of a number of different kinds of intelligence which include intellectual, verbal, social, practical and personal. Although they feel that emotional intelligence generally operates as a unitary phenomenon, four separate elements can be recognized (Salovey and Mayer 1990, Mayer and Salovey 1997, Mayer et al 2000). This is now known as the four-branch model which proceeds from perception to management:

- The perception and expression of emotion in the self and others.
- The use of emotion to facilitate thought, and the integration of emotion in thought.

- Understanding and analysing emotions in self and others.
- Regulating and managing emotions in self and others depending on one's needs, goals and plans (the management of relationships).

In his helpful paper introducing the concept of emotional intelligence to social workers, Morrison (2007: 251), along with Gardner (1993), also recognizes that two of these domains are *intra*personal (self-awareness and self-management), and two are *inter*personal (awareness of others and relationship skills), but, of course, there is a relationship between the two. Self-awareness affects the ability of the individual to be aware of the emotional condition of others. The ability to regulate your own emotions affects the skill with which you are able to manage your dealings and relationship with others.

Our days are suffused with emotional content. We feel embarrassed when we make a fool of ourselves in public, we follow the emotional ups and downs of the characters in 'soaps', we become lost in romantic fiction, we frighten ourselves watching horror films. We rarely reflect on the emotional twists and turns of everyday life. Mayer and Salovey (1997) see us bobbing through each day on a river of unbidden emotion, most of which seems on reflection to be trivial and yet emotions occupy so much of daily life. We worry, feel angry, become excited, get frustrated. Here, a social worker is thinking about the day ahead:

I know I'm putting off writing the conclusion and making recommendations in the Sharpley case, and I know why. I suppose I think at one level the two young children should be adopted, but I keep surprising myself by feeling sorry for Mrs Sharpley. She's had a shit awful life, full of pain and rejection and violent, useless partners and I have to sympathise. The psychiatrist says that she has an antisocial personality disorder. She's certainly aggressive and intimidating with everyone, including the children – and I do worry about them and how they're being affected by her parenting. The health visitor said she has to really steel herself before she can make a home visit which I can totally understand. I feel relieved now that my interview with Mrs Sharpley is over. She's rubbished me, threatened me, apologised, broken down in tears saying she can't bear to live without the kids and that's left me feeling confused, rotten and knotted up inside. I know that this is not the time to make a rash judgement, particularly when one minute I'm feeling hostile and punitive, and then the next I'm chillingly aware of the enormity of the decision to remove the children leaving her with nothing. The sickening pain I know I would feel if someone took my children off me would be impossible to bear. Alice is in the office today but I won't discuss the case with her. She will only get excited and outraged and make me feel stupid for even thinking about any option other than removal and eventual adoption. I'll sleep on it overnight, if I can sleep, and wait until Joanne is back. She knows how this case churns me up but she'll help me understand what's going on a whole lot better than Alice.

Emotions can arise suddenly and with the surprising ability to take up so much immediate mental space. Small trains of thought appear, driven by one emotion only to be overtaken by another a short while later. Emotional intelligence occurs in those able to recognize and take cognisance, if not control of this froth of feeling that covers so much of the psychological content of our days.

From Monitoring to Management

We can recognize six elements in the make-up of emotionally intelligent people. Emotionally intelligent individuals:

- are aware of and monitor their emotions;
- register and provide feedback on other people's emotions;
- use emotion to improve their reasoning;
- understand and analyse their own and other people's affective states;
- regulate and manage their own and other people's emotions and arousal; and
- co-operate and collaborate with others in mutually rewarding relationships.

Let's look at these elements in more details.

(1) Emotionally intelligent people are aware of and *monitor their emotions*, particularly emotions that have a strong affect on perception,

behaviour, thought and understanding. For example, although John might have a soft spot for Emma, what she has just said about Mary, who can be irritating, is unnecessarily sarcastic and unfair, particularly as Mary, to his surprise, has made an interesting point. John feels uncomfortable but decides that if the discussion is to return to more constructive ground, Emma's cutting remark and Mary's wounded reaction need a diplomatic and resolving comment from him. Emotionally intelligent men and women also realize that we can have multiple, contrasting, even conflicting emotions. A person may feel anxious at the prospect of giving a public speech, but also a little excited and thrilled. John likes Emma but is cross with her for being so rude and unhelpful. Novelists, of course, have a knack of capturing emotional matters much better than dry academics. Here is a nice example of someone able to acknowledge that emotions can conflict given by the author (and part time journalist and agony aunt), Virginia Ironside as we enter the diary reflections of the novel's principal character Marie Sharp:

> I remember only recently realizing that you could hold two feelings in yourself at the same time, that you could both like someone and dislike them in one go . . . As one who sees life rather in black and white – strong hates and loves – I have always tried to compromise by seeing everything in a kind of grey. The trick is not to do that at all, but to hold the contrasts in oneself at exactly the same time. That results in a much more lively and invigorating approach. Very late in the day to discover that thought, but it has made relationships with people far, far easier. And oddly, kinder. (Ironside 2007: 11)

(2) Emotionally intelligent individuals register, note, interpret, reflect and provide feed back on *other people's emotions* as they are expressed in their faces, voices, gestures, movements. Emotionally intelligent people *listen*. They are *empathic*. It is also recognized that inner emotional states might not always correspond with a person's outward expression – that a smile might hide pain, that a laugh might mask anxiety. Or that one's own behaviour and emotional expressions may affect someone else's feelings. We need therefore to be not only aware how we present ourselves emotionally but how this might affect other people. And beyond mutual emotional awareness,

there is a higher level in which we feel able to share our feelings in the safety of a secure, intimate relationship with a lover, close friend, respected colleague.

(3) Emotionally intelligent people *use emotion to improve their reasoning*. If we are reflectively aware of our emotions, we can 'capture the wisdom of our feelings' (Hein 2006: 4). Emotions affect what we think, how we think and what we do. For example, happiness tends to make us more positive in our outlook. When we are feeling good, we feel more positive about other people. Happiness can make us more creative, more co-operative and well-disposed to our fellows. The pioneering work of Isen illustrates this effect with particular elegance. In a series of experiments, she induced feelings of mild happiness and pleasure in subjects who then went on to appraise and interact with the world more positively (eg Isen and Levin 1972; Isen et al 1991). If someone offers you a kindness (for example, lets you join the busy traffic on the highway from a side road), you, in turn, are more likely to be courteous to other motorists, at least for a short while. Success in one aspect of one's job (eg praise from a colleague) can make you more effective in another (more thorough and accurate assessments of the needs of those who use your services). In general, emotionally intelligent people are better problem-solvers, motivators and team leaders. They are more likely to be flexible and creative thinkers.

Managers and team leaders are well advised to take note of these findings. Emotionally intelligent people not only create positive and constructive feeling states in themselves, they are also gifted in bringing about similar states in those around them. Conversely, negative emotions make us less productive, less creative, and more awkward with others. In many areas of life, including those which are creative or interpersonal, thought is enhanced by feeling. Emotions can help put thoughts in order giving some ideas and plans higher priority than others.

We also recognize that emotions can disrupt our thoughts. Anxiety upsets our thinking. When we are stressed we feel we can't concentrate, we can't think straight.

In general, emotions give 'valence' – either negative or positive – to experience (Mayer et al 2000: 107). In this sense feelings colour memory; they shade the value we give to a person, an object, an event. Meeting a difficult father after we have just suffered a set-back in court not only increases the chance that the interview might not go well, the father is also more likely to be cast in a negative light simply because the interview was stressful. It takes a special effort to think about the father rationally and objectively and without emotional distortion. Individuals who can reflect on their own mental processes and what drives them tend to be socially skilled. They don't ignore or even try to control their emotions. Rather, they are able to use their feelings as valuable information that guides the conduct of the relationship.

(4) Emotionally intelligent people therefore *understand and analyse their own and other people's affective states*, particularly as they colour social interaction. They are aware of the origin and cause of their current emotional condition and how this is affecting their thoughts and behaviour. Those who are able to recognize the origins and causes of emotional states and how they affect the self and others display higher levels of emotional intelligence. They also understand that different, even conflicting emotions can co-exist or that one feeling can lead to another, and that in the matters of arousal and feeling, there is a swirl and a momentum in which emotions appear to take on a life of their own. Those who are quick to blame fate or external events for how they feel are not showing emotional intelligence. Passively allowing yourself to be tossed around by powerful feelings or impersonal destiny shows a lack of emotional curiosity and cognitive resolve.

The challenge is to recognize and understand how what happens to us makes feel the way we do. This can be difficult and salutary. It can be uncomfortable, for example, to admit that it was really envy and jealousy that made you behave so aggressively towards the man who got early promotion. This is not to say that external affairs do not need attention or change, but rather to be wise about how, when and why we feel the way we do. Emotions do not just arise out of nowhere. Our history, our make-up, our circumstances are all involved. We really must fight against seeing ourselves as passive in the face of arousal and feeling. We need to know ourselves and most especially our emotional selves.

Emotional understanding is therefore used for social problem-solving. Mayer, Salovey and Caruso (2000) have developed measures for different components of emotional intelligence. They comprise the Multifactor Emotional Intelligence Scale or MEIS. An example of an item on the MEIS asks the respondent to decide which two emotions best define 'contempt':

Contempt most closely combines which two emotions:

1. anger and fear
2. fear and surprise
3. disgust and anger
4. surprise and disgust

[The correct answer is 3 – disgust and anger]

The MEIS, and other similar measures, typically contain many such questions, each testing a particular component of emotional intelligence. Sometimes a short story is presented and the respondent is asked about some aspect of the emotional make-up of the situation (Taylor and Bagby 2000):

Instructions: In this part, you will read a story and indicate the emotions which you believe the person telling the story was feeling. This story comes from an 11 year old girl:

I don't feel like practising the violin. My dad said that I have to, but then he asked me to do something else. That's good, because I hate to practise. I'll do the other chore my dad asked me to do so that I can delay practising my violin. My brother plays piano but my parents don't make him practise like I have to.

	Definitely NOT present				Definitely PRESENT
Anger	1	2	3	4	5
Happy	1	2	3	4	5
Fearful	1	2	3	4	5
Surprised	1	2	3	4	5
Sad	1	2	3	4	5

Another common measure involves the presentation of a photo-graph in which someone is expressing an emotion, or two or more people are engaged with each other over some matter (it could be an argument, an apology by one to the other, a shared disappointment). The respondent is asked what emotions are likely to be present.

A particularly interesting exercise to measure empathy has been devised by Baron-Cohen et al (2001): The 'Reading the Mind in the Eyes' test. The person being tested is shown a series of 36 faces, each expressing a different emotion, but with only the eyes showing. The eyes, of course, are the most emotionally expressive bit of our faces. Four possible answers are given for each picture. For example, the respondent might be given four options for a 'look in the eyes' that expresses a thoughtful, pensive mood. The respondent is asked which of the four words they think best describes what the person in the picture is thinking or feeling: (i) irritated, (ii) pensive, (iii) hostile, or (iv) excited. On average women tend to score better than men on this test, although it has to be noted that being only an average some men do perform extremely well while some women turn out to be rather poor emotional empathisers. People with autism and Asperger Syndrome also score less well. Children who have suffered neglect are also at risk of being poor emotional mind readers. Children who have suffered physical abuse are good at interpreting angry facial expressions, though less skilled at differentiating other emotions including fear, surprise and even happiness.

I have carried out a similar teaching exercise to gauge people's emotional awareness. I show a video clip of a soap opera, TV drama or documentary of a couple in counselling – with the sound turned off. I then ask the class to guess what is happening and just go 'with their gut feelings' – what is the issue, what are the characters feeling and why, what is the dialogue about? It is surprising how uncannily accurate some people are in sensing what is taking place.

(5) Emotionally intelligent people are able to *regulate and manage their own and other people's emotions and arousal.* They achieve this by being aware of their own feelings and reflecting on what they might mean. 'This ability comprises the most advanced skills, ranging from the ability to stay open to feelings – both pleasant and unpleasant ones – to the ability to manage emotions in oneself and others by enhancing pleasant ones and moderating negative ones' (Neubauer and Freudenthaler 2005: 36). Mayer (2001) believes that 'management

of emotion begins with being open to emotion. If emotions are informative, then opening oneself to such information will enable one to know more about the surrounding world – particularly the world of relationships – than if one were closed . . . Only by perceiving and understanding emotions can one understand the outcomes of experiencing them or cutting them off' (p 422).

Those who are good at managing emotions tend to choose effective emotional responses in complex social situations. A social care worker learns that she cannot provide a particular service that she knows an older person was hoping to receive. The last time she was in a similar situation, the service user made a complaint. The care worker knows the next home visit is going to be uncomfortable but has not yet fully acknowledged that this is the emotionally charged reason for putting off the interview. The longer she delays the visit, the more agitated she feels and this distressed mood begins to affect the rest of her work including the desire to come into work. One evening she puts together all these emotional pieces, takes a deep breath, and knows that she will actually feel better the sooner she gets on with breaking the unwelcome news to 83 year old Mrs Ellis. She realizes that the feelings of diffuse agitation are actually less pleasant than the prospect of making the home visit.

(6) Emotionally intelligent people integrate all the above skills and so demonstrate their *ability to co-operate, collaborate and co-construct mutually rewarding and successful relationships*. These affective talents are particularly useful when working or socializing in a group context. Emotionally intelligent people are good at negotiation and resolving conflicts. They are able to provide and receive emotional closeness, care and concern. We tend to enjoy their company. People are drawn to them at times of need.

The Personal and Interpersonal Benefits of Emotional Intelligence

Emotionally intelligent people are able to self-motivate and persist even when the going gets tough. Emotions are harnessed so that attention is kept, tasks are pursued, focus is maintained. Emotionally competent individuals respond creatively when faced with tricky social situations. They are social problem-solvers.

These talents can be spotted at surprisingly young ages. Two groups of five year olds are each given a toy telescope. One group squabbles and fights over who gets to look down the telescope. After five minutes no-one in the group has had a proper chance to peer through the instrument. The other group also begins by fighting over the telescope, but after a minute a young girl, Zelda, makes a suggestion. 'Let's all take equal turns. Jack, you go first, then Emma, then Ali and then me. Is that OK?' The group immediately agrees. The resolution of the potential conflict by Zelda is particularly smart as Jack and Emma are clearly more impatient to have a turn than either Ali or the girl herself. After five minutes all four children have had a good view. Jack and Emma are quickly bored with the telescope, leaving Ali and Zelda with as much time as they want to play with the device.

Reviewing these emotional strengths, Saarni (2000) believes that collectively they lead to:

> . . . *skill in managing one's emotions*, which is critical to being able to negotiate one's way through interpersonal exchanges. Other important consequences of emotional competence are *a sense of subjective well-being* and adaptive *resilience* in the face of future stressful circumstances' (p 78, emphasis original)

As we have seen, the long term benefits of emotional intelligence can be identified as early as the first few years of life. Mischel and his colleagues (cited in Shoda et al 1990) observed that impulsive four year olds who find it difficult to delay gratification, who fail to see any potential benefit in waiting even when told that patience will bring greater rewards (for example, being told 'you can have a piece of chocolate now or if you wait 10 minutes, you'll get twice as much chocolate') are at increased risk as adolescents of a range of problem behaviours, mental health concerns and educational underachievement. The children who did manage to wait and contain their desire (and thus receive twice as much chocolate) enjoyed much brighter prospects. In adolescence, they possessed higher levels of social skill and emotional intelligence. They were also more likely to be performing well at school. And ten or years more after the delayed gratification experiment, they were still able to control their impulses and pursue desired goals more successfully. For example, they were willing to study hard for success or save pocket money to buy a new bike.

Goleman (1995) cites the findings of the early years pre-school project, *Head Start (The Emotional Foundations of School Readiness)*, which found that so much of school success depends on emotional intelligence: 'being self-assured and interested; knowing what kind of behaviour is expected and how to rein in the impulse to misbehave; being able to wait, to follow directions, and to turn to teachers for help; and expressing need while getting along with other children' (Goleman 1995: 194; Brazelton 1992). The successful children showed early confidence in the availability and likely helpfulness of adults. The children appeared curious about and fascinated by new experiences which they approached positively and with pleasure. 'They knew *how* to learn' writes Goleman (1995: 194). They displayed good social understanding. Without sacrificing their own needs and goals, they were socially co-operative. They had the ability to communicate their own ideas, feelings, plans and concepts.

Working Under Stress

There is certainly the strong message that those graced with emotional intelligence will probably set about life positively and enjoy relationships. In this sense, they are less likely to meet stress but if they do have to deal with challenge and pressure, they are likely to cope well. Emotional intelligence therefore has close links with the 'coping and stress' literature. It suggests resilience. And as stress is associated with the increased risk of dysfunctional behaviour and poor mental and physical health, emotional intelligence may act as a major protective factor for both social workers and service users as they face situations that are stressful. Therefore helping people develop and improve their emotional intelligence is likely to be of benefit.

Stress increases anxiety and anxiety makes rational thought and action more difficult. When we experience anxiety, our mental energy and defences are consumed by the feelings of distress. We can't concentrate. At such times, we fail to connect with other people. As a result we are less collaborative and unable to co-operate constructively. This lack of affective attunement and cognitive connection reduces the professional's emotional availability, effectiveness and value. Similarly, service users under stress also lose the ability to remain emotionally attuned. They find that relationships become more volatile and conflictual, or lifeless and empty. This upsets marriages, undermines parenting, and leads to anti-social behaviour. Service users under stress can be accused by professionals of being resistant and unco-operative. In contrast, emotionally intelligent workers will want to think about why the user is behaving so aggressively or feeling so anxious. Understanding the origins of the anger and anxiety and what triggers such feelings not only leads to more intelligent management of the service user's arousal, but it might also provide clues about how best to tackle the underlying issues.

Service users under stress are likely to make professionals feel stressed. At such times, the professional-user relationship is in danger of breaking down. The emotionally intelligent social worker has to be particularly aware of her or his own feelings and defences on such occasions. And although heightened emotions are a time when relationships can run into trouble, when handled well, times of stress and strong feeling can also lead to great personal learning. The skilled practitioner uses the rawness of powerful, negative emotions to help those in pain and angry despair recognize, reflect on and regulate their potentially destructive feelings. This is only possible if the professional has the emotional intelligence and skill to contain the other at times when they feel emotionally adrift and out-of-control.

Conclusion

Emotional intelligence has risen rapidly up the agenda of most health and social care professionals. In practice, it is less a body of knowledge and more a knowledge of how our bodies, minds and relationships work at the level of emotions and feeling. But what are emotions and why do we have them? Answers to these questions plunge us into an exotic mix of evolutionary theory, human physiology, neurobiology, and developmental and social psychology.

3
What are Emotions?

Introduction

One way of asking what emotions are is to examine their evolution-ary and biological origins. We are then forced to ask a number of supplementary questions: Why do have feelings? What are emotions for? And why do human beings in particular have such an extraordi-nary range of emotional states? In this chapter we consider the evolu-tionary advantages that emotions appear to confer on most group living species, particularly human beings, the value of emotions in social problem-solving, and how feelings affect both mind and body.

In Body and Mind

In the 1980s, psychology became interested in evolutionary theory. Evolutionary theorists are keen to know what is the adaptive value of any genetic trait, physiological feature, species-specific behaviour or general attribute. Psychologists began to apply an evolutionary perspective to human thought, feeling and behaviour. They began to ask questions. For example, how and why did we acquire language? What was the adaptive value of long term memory? Why do we have emotions? What's their function? Superficially we all know what emotions are and can probably name dozens of them quite quickly. But a moment's reflection suggests that at both a descriptive and scientific level they are rather curious, complex and not a little elusive.

Interestingly, it was Charles Darwin who first addressed the ques-tion of emotions and their place in our evolutionary history. In 1872 he wrote *The Expression of the Emotions in Man and Animals*. The book introduced a revolutionary new way of thinking about emotion. Darwin was interested in the way animals and humans express emotional states in terms of their physiology and behaviour. In particular, he felt that facial expressions offered a window into the inner world of our minds.

Darwin identified the principal emotions in terms of how they are expressed and how the body behaves. We ache with loss. Feelings of shame, he observed, result in blushing and a dilation of blood vessels on the face and in the neck. When we feel angry, the heart beats faster pumping blood to the muscles and limbs in readiness for a *fight* response. As the blood flows faster, so the skin reddens and we feel hot. Fear also triggers an increase in adrenaline and heart rate, but here blood, carrying oxygen and energy, is directed to the long muscles to aid escape and *flight*. Blood drains away from the body's surface where it's not needed, leaving the skin feeling cold, and so we 'shiver with fear.' All movement freezes as our senses are in state of heightened alert. Surprise also demands that we pay attention. The eyes open wide and the eyebrows raise in order to take in as much visual information as possible so that we might take quick stock of the unexpected situation. In contrast, when we feel happy and loving, our bodies feel calm and content, our minds feel engaged, and we approach others in a spirit of friendship and co-operation. In short, each emotion seems to prepare the body for a certain type of response. Emotions take place in the body as much as they do in the mind.

The recognition that emotions have (i) subjective, (ii) expressive, and (iii) behavioural aspects provides an important and early clue that the emotions have to be understood at a number of interconnected levels. They affect the *mind*, they animate the *face*, and they arouse the *body*. We read people's emotional condition by noting the look on their face, interpreting their body language, listening to what they say and how they say it. These links between the mind and the body turn out to be extremely important in trying to understand the nature and power of the emotions. Our everyday language certainly captures these states. We say we are 'consumed with fear'. Someone's tears are inconsolable. We talk of feeling helpless with laughter. Indeed, emotionally intelligent people appear to use this understanding of how the emotions affect the body, in themselves and others, as useful social and psychological knowledge.

And when a feeling persists for hours, days or weeks we talk of being in a certain 'mood'. Curiously, we use colour to describe many of our moods and feelings. When we are depressed we speak of feeling blue. Green is the colour of envy, yellow the colour of cowardice. Those in a 'brown study' are said to be in thoughtful and contemplative mood. When we feel bright, cheerful and healthy we are 'in the pink'. And behind brooding menace lie dark thoughts and black feelings.

Colour is also used by designers to affect our mood. A psychology of colour has arisen to support these ideas. In moderation, red can energize us. It makes us feel more vital, more passionate. It stimulates our appetites for food, drink and sex. But in excess, too much red makes us feel anxious, even irritable. Rooms coloured green – the dominant colour in nature – can make us feel calm and in balance. Light blues have been associated with serenity. Sky blues relax us. However as few foods are coloured blue, it has been suggested that appetites are suppressed when walls are painted cobalt or sapphire. Black can induce feelings of power and convey elegance but when overdone it can feel oppressive and threatening. Yellow, the colour of the sun, makes us cheerful, even inventive. Colours also convey messages to other people. White is worn for purity and innocence of thought and feeling. We dress in grey to suggest a sober and serious attitude. Red clothes are for fun, raciness and even danger.

These metaphorical and literal uses of colour to describe feelings, induce mood and suggest character hint at the links between the senses and our emotions. It may be that if we are to understand human nature in terms of the relationship between mind and body, the senses and our psychology have to be thought about not as two separate realms but connected and highly integrated. It is yet another reminder that emotions are experienced both physiologically and psychologically giving them an immediate, earthy quality as well as a more cerebral character.

Negative Emotions

In general, emotions lead to either an *approach* or *avoidance* response with the more negative emotions leading to escape and avoidance behaviours. There are in fact far more negative emotions than positive. Again, from an evolutionary perspective this makes sense. Survival is the bottom line for any individual member of a species. Anything that threatens our survival, including social and personal rejection, is likely to make us feel agitated or uncomfortable. '[E]volution appears to have been more interested in keeping us alive than making us happy. Overall, negative emotions trump positive ones and weigh more heavily in our evaluation of people and situa-tion' (Cozolino 2006: 318). There are many ways in which to be miserable, but relatively few in which to be happy. 'All happy fami-lies resemble one another', wrote Tolstoy (1875/2003), 'but each unhappy family is unhappy in its own way'.

Fear, shame, disgust, embarrassment, terror, jealousy, and anger are examples of *negative emotions* that we try to do something about once we experience them. We might reduce feelings of fear by escap-ing to a safe place. We might try to deal with shame by trying to conform to group expectations and not stepping outside social norms and 'making a fool of ourselves'. Jealousy may force us to let go of a relationship that is no longer a source of pleasure and is now only a cause of hurt and pain. In each case, the emotion is felt both in the body and the mind. And in each case, the emotion leads to some kind of action the purpose of which is to reduce the negative feeling and get us into a different place, either physically, psychologically or socially.

Anger occurs when the passage of a positive emotion is thwarted and blocked. Anger can lead to attack behaviour in an attempt to recover the object, resource or situation. We attempt to assert ourselves as more demanding and dominant. Anger can also make us more determined to achieve what is resisting our best efforts. More generally, when we are in a negative mood we feel less co-operative, helpful and responsive. We are also likely to judge people and prod-ucts less favourably. But anger is not always negative in its outcome. It can lead to discussion, negotiation, resolution and recovery when protagonists feel that their new agreed position is more open and healthy and they can both move on. Certainly in close relationships, there is evidence that modicums of anger are not as threatening to the viability of the relationship as are withdrawal, contempt or disin-terest (eg Jenkins et al 1989; Gottman and Levenson 1992).

Contempt occurs when there is angry rejection of someone else. It tends to lead to separation of those involved, whether partners in a marriage or people within a group. Once separated, they get on with their lives and might never meet again. However, there are many occasions when feelings of contempt arise but it is not easy for those involved to part. This can apply to individuals as well as cultural, ethnic and religious groups who are geographically bound together.

People are capable of cruel and violent behaviour towards those for whom they feel nothing but contempt, believing them to be 'less than human' and deserving of hurt and humiliation. In this sense, contempt and hatred are some of the most dangerous and destructive emotions. In diminishing the humanity of the other, they can lead to violence, murder and elimination. In these cases, contempt and verbal abuse are an attempt to place the other outside of what is accepted, to put them beyond the pale, diminished and alone. To be outside 'society' or the group and be alone is a dangerous place in which to be.

Disgust is felt when an object provokes feelings of revulsion. In evolutionary terms, rotting meats, faeces, infected wounds, and foods with a nauseating smell indicate danger to health. Feelings of disgust lead to the avoidance of contaminating and ill-making objects. By extension, people and their nauseous and noxious behaviour, can also bring about feelings of disgust if their actions appear to taint and spoil what we value and uphold.

Positive Feelings

Positive feelings are those we have when we are drawn to approach and stay with an experience that is to our benefit. Love, joy and happiness are pleasurable states in which to be. They keep us involved and connected. They facilitate romance and courtship, mating, marriage, parenting, caregiving, co-operation, group cohesion, and friendship. As very social animals, humans feel most safe and relaxed when they are accepted members of a group. The group might be based on the family, community, work, or play. Danger is experienced when we are apart from the group, when we are on our own. Thus, loss, rejection and abandonment by others cause feelings that are troubling, feelings that are primitive in their power because they operate at a deep biological level, a level that speaks of our very existence and survival.

Feeling happy and content keeps us engaged and absorbed in what we are doing. Feeling happy also tends to make us more co-operative, helpful, generous, confident, receptive, responsive, flexible, decisive, expansive, inclusive and creative (Forgas 2001b). Emotions that occur along the axis of love and affection are key to understanding our ability to work together as a species and stay together in collaborative partnerships over time. Marriages, long term friendships, and parent–child bonds endure when there is pleasure to be found in the relationship.

We also tend to judge people, arguments and products more favourably when we are in a positive mood. People in good moods are more likely to think they are enjoying good health or that the economy is improving. In contrast, negative emotions cause us to stop or depart from what we are doing. People in a poor state of mind describe themselves as suffering poorer health and have a more pessimistic outlook on the economy.

Emotions and Memory

The more emotionally significant, unique and life-changing the experience, the more it is likely to be remembered. Although you might have driven to work on countless occasions without remembering any journey in particular, the day that someone crashed into you causing a serious cut and scar on your right hand, that journey and the details surrounding the accident will be remembered. Or the time when you felt deeply embarrassed by your behaviour in an important social gathering will also be recalled vividly many years later. The effect of an emotionally charged event is that it is both more likely to be remembered and remembered in better detail than an emotionally less significant event.

It is also the case that we tend to remember things better that resonate with our current mood. If we are feeling sad, sad memories seem easier to recall. When we are in a happy mood, more positive memories seem to surface more readily. The advantage of this affectively selective remembering is that we can access memories and actions that resonate with our current mood so they help guide our current behaviour in the similarly emotionally coloured situation.

Environment of Evolutionary Adaptedness

Darwin weaved his thinking about the emotions into his theory of evolution. He saw the emotions as basic but effective. Their nature and origins have to be understood in terms of the value they conferred on ancient issues of survival and adaptation. For example, a sneer of contempt is little more than the snarl of aggression. Like many other mammals, our hair bristles when we experience sudden fear and terror. We suffer embarrassment when we act foolishly, shame when we fail in the context of a group, and experience surprise when something unexpected happens. Emotions, both at the physiological and psychological level, create feelings that sweep over us and through us whether we like it or not. And being basic, when they first arise, emotions are largely out of conscious control. Nevertheless, they have function; they have value.

As animals interact with their environment, they constantly encounter problems and opportunities. In our 'environments of evolutionary adaptedness', many of these encounters are literally matters of life and death. When to run away, when to fight. What to eat, what not to eat. Who to approach, who to avoid. At stake is the individual's survival and ability to reproduce. 'Emotions evolved as solutions to such perennial problems and opportunities. Different kinds of problems and opportunities made necessary different adaptive behaviours' (Stemmler 2004: 34). Kitayama et al (2004) suggest that 'emotions may best be seen as nature's way to help the self navigate in uncertain terrains of daily social life in more or less adaptive ways. According to this view emotions serve as indispensable "pathfinders" for the self' (p 252). So, for example, the basic emotions sponsor particular behavioural patterns:

> . . . one prompts continuation with current activity when things are going well (happiness), another prompts giving up and backtracking when there has been loss (sadness), another prompts aggression when a goal is blocked (anger), another prompts freezing and paying attention to dangers in the environment when a threat occurs (fear). (Oatley 1998: 287)

Over evolutionary time, the link between these problems, opportunities and adaptive solutions led to quick, automatic responses that involved both body and mind. Each problem, each opportunity evolved into a particular emotion. Each emotion excites us to feel and act in a unique way under set conditions. Each emotion is therefore a brain/body state that is activated in response to an environmental event that represents a chance or challenge.

Emotions appear initially to operate outside immediate consciousness. A feature of the environment is first experienced via one or more of the senses. The experience may pose danger or conflict or an opportunity. The body and the emotional centres of the brain react to the experience by rapidly preparing the individual for a fast, appropriate response. Fear triggers a flight response. Removal of a desired object and conflict are likely to lead to anger. An opportunity brings feelings of excitement and pleasure. Evolutionists believe that these fast responses happen before the individual is able consciously to reflect on the experience. Although emotional reactions lack subtlety, they are quick and powerful and thus they provide individuals with a large number of immediate, automatic, in-built, adaptive, non-reflective behavioural responses.

In contrast to feeling, thinking is relatively slow. If you had to think about and evaluate a potential danger or threat or mating opportunity, you might end up either dead or a reproductive failure. Evolutionary theorists recognize the value of emotions in terms of survival and reproduction. In this sense, emotions are largely instinctive reactions to certain kinds of stimuli.

> Emotions are the result of complex neural mechanisms that show all the hallmarks of special design. They are, in other words, adaptations designed by natural selection ... [and] a creature that lacked all emotional capacities simply could not survive. (Evans and Cruse 2004: xii)

Emotions, believes Goleman (1995: xii), are impulses to act: we approach or avoid, we attack or defend. These emotion systems 'can be seen as time-tested solutions to timeless problems and challenges' (Levenson 2003 cited in Stemmler 2004: 34). Emotions process information to dangers and opportunities not yet experienced. What they do is rapidly orientate us to do something about the experience when we do actually meet it. Affective behaviours therefore regulate behaviour *in the absence of prior experience*. Our emotions, says Goleman (1995), 'guide us in facing predicaments and tasks too important to leave to intellect alone' (p 4). This is why when we are in an aroused emotional state, what we see, what we think, and how we behave are deeply influenced by that emotion. Emotions ensure that we pay attention to the things that matter until the matter is dealt with.

In their review of the work of the evolutionists Tooby and Cosmides (1990), Oatley and Jenkins (1996) neatly sum up the evolutionary base of the emotions noting that:

Emotions arise largely with problems to be solved. So for recurring problems like escaping from predators, responding to strangers, meeting aggressive threats, caring for infants, falling in love, and so on, we are equipped with genetically based mechanisms that provide outline scripts for behaviour that has been successful in the past, and therefore has been selected. Each kind of emotional pattern is triggered by distinctive cues. Each makes ready patterns of action appropriate to solving the problem that has arisen. (p 82)

It therefore seems reasonable to assume that our emotions evolved to suit the physical and social environment in which our species developed. There is general agreement that the early evolutionary history of human beings probably occurred in East Africa at least 250,000 years ago. The environment to which our species had to adapt was one of relatively open landscapes and coastlines. Our ancient ancestors lived in small, hunter-gatherer groups.

If these social groups were to function as complex, collaborative units, it would have been necessary to establish co-operation and cohesion between members. Human beings are social beings and group living is fundamental to survival. In groups we co-operate, create and share resources. We experience strength in numbers. We therefore feel safe when we are part of the family and social group. In the evolutionary past, these small communities were the source of food, safety and protection. Even in the modern socially complex world, if we are to function competently, at work, play or during courtship, we need to be able to negotiate relationships, groups and social hierarchies.

It is also the case that at birth and for the first few years of life, human infants are highly vulnerable and dependent. Without the care of their mothers and other adults, babies simply would not survive. This is probably why any sense of abandonment by caregivers, or rejection by the group causes us such anxiety and fear. Abandonment, whether physical or psychological, triggers very strong feelings of alarm and anxiety. To be alone and outside the group, or to be abandoned, deliberately or accidentally, by one's parents are extremely hazardous and *feared* states in which to be. These highly distressing feelings echo throughout our social life making us particularly sensitive to any hint of rejection, disinterest or loss by those to whom we feel close, reliant and dependent.

As human infants remain dependent for many years, it is in the genetic interest of both mothers and fathers to ensure as much stability and security as possible if the child is to reach reproductive age. From an evolutionary perspective, there is therefore an incentive for both parents to remain together, at least for several years until the child becomes independent. Emotions that help maintain romantic attachments between parents and sustain strong caregiving bonds between parents and child improve the survival chances of infants. Feelings of love keep parents together and mothers and babies bonded and attached.

Species that do not rear their young have little need of the emotions of love and affection, sadness and regret. Most female fish simply release eggs into the water which then get fertilised by male sperm. In the absence of parents, the eggs are left to hatch. Once born, the very small, young fish are on their own. There is no parental awareness, interest or involvement in their subsequent fate. The story is similar for most reptiles and amphibians. Once their eggs are laid, parent frogs and turtles have no further relationship with their young, or indeed their sexual mate. They have no behavioural instincts to nurture or protect their progeny. Feelings of love (and loss) that sponsor bonds and attachment are simply not present. They're not necessary. Therefore those parts of the brain that deal with and process our emotions and their experience remain underdeveloped in amphibians and reptiles. All of this being the case, the faces of fish, frogs and snakes are relatively expressionless. They have few emotions which to express and no need to express them.

For human beings, any behaviour that enhances social bonding increases an individual's chances of survival and ability to reproduce. If emotions are woven into the individual's experience of social relationships such that bonding, approval and acceptance feel good, while separation, devaluation and rejection feel bad, then we begin to see the part that emotions might play in human intercourse. If one of the defining characteristics of human beings is their social competence and ability to co-operate, these elements are first found in the loving, trusting relationship between vulnerable, dependent infants and their responsive, protective caregivers.

In terms of evolution, very little time has passed between our early nomadic hunter-gatherer roots and modern 21st century life. The emotions that arose in response to the 'environment of evolutionary adaptedness' (Bowlby 1969) are still present with all their force and potency, but are now played out in the buzz of our highly complex urban, technological and densely populated societies. Emotions fast track us into a more energetic, albeit simple actions and behavioural responses. 'What evolution has equipped us with, therefore, is a set of emotional states that organize ready repertoires of action' (Oatley and Jenkins 1996: 258). They may be relatively crude in character but because of the adaptive nature of their evolutionary genesis, the actions that emotions prompt have a greater chance of being behaviourally effective. Emotions help us to cope with the unexpected twists and turns of day-to-day relationships. They provoke quick, unconscious actions and reactions. They give us rapid solutions to the problems generated by the fast flow of social life. 'Emotions' writes Oatley (2004: 4), 'give life its urgency'.

Expressing Emotions

Because we are a social, group living species, it makes evolutionary sense to be able to read each other's intentions and behaviour, thoughts and feelings. Emotions help structure social relationships. They act as an in-built social compass that tells us when to approach, back off, become more intimate, assert, apologize, make amends. Human beings have a very complex facial musculature and we use most of these muscles to express feeling. We can configure our faces to express a wide range of emotions the most basic and universal of which are fear, happiness, sadness, anger, surprise, and disgust. These universal emotions are also known as the primary emotions.

Ekman's (1989) pioneering research established that nearly all cultures recognize the meaning and significance of each of these basic feelings. We recognize the same emotional expressions on the faces of those from very different parts of the world. The happy face of a tribesman from Polynesia is recognized as the expression of joy by people whether they live in London, New York, Rio de Janeiro, Calcutta, Shanghai or Lagos. So, although different cultures give more or less social weight to particular emotions and may have unique conventions about their expression, the universal feelings of happiness, anger, sadness, disgust, fear, and surprise appear shared, recognized and understood by all humanity. It therefore seems reasonable to suggest that we are all born with the same genetic emotional template, although our feelings become subtly refined, elaborated and differentiated as we grow and develop in our own familial and cultural setting (Oatley and Jenkins 1996: 50).

Many of our facial expressions are reflexes. They are in-built and automatic reactions to a given stimulus, typically a social stimulus. Such expressions convey information to others about our feelings and intentions. They signal our mental state. They set the tone for social interaction. A smile is encouraging and facilitative. A look of suspicion indicates caution and wariness, or even a lack of trust. Eyebrows fleetingly raised convey recognition, and in some cases, particularly if repeated quickly in sequence, might be interpreted as flirtation. Facial expressions convey an awful lot of social and emotional information without a word ever being uttered. Again, this reminds us that the emotions have their origins deep within our pre-lingual evolutionary history, and what they might lack in sophistication they make up in power and directness. Even deaf-and-blind children show a wide variety of facial expressions and body postures to suggest feelings of happiness or distress, surprise or distaste, albeit displayed in less refined and nuanced ways than hearing and sighted children (Eibl-Eibesfeldt 1973).

We therefore communicate our interior mental states through facial expression, body posture and vocalisation. 'This communication provides others with information about one's likely behavioral intentions and gives them some extra time to adapt accordingly before one's own behavioral actions are actually launched' (Stemmler 2004: 35). Emotional expression helps in the smooth running of groups as each member reads, interprets and adjusts his or her own behaviour in order to stay safe but also maximize opportunities, connect with others and also ensure one's own needs are met. For example, we tend to show deference when we are in the company of those whom we perceive as more dominant, powerful and who possess key resources. When we meet those who are weak and vulnerable, we tend to respond protectively and with nurturance, although a few individuals, particularly those who are very uncertain about their own social value, might react more aggressively or exploitatively.

Our ability to empathize with other people's feelings is also largely based on our skill in interpreting their facial expressions. The eyes in particular seem to say a lot about our emotional condition.

As we saw in Chapter Two, experiments by Baron-Cohen (2004) have shown that even when people are shown only the eyes of someone expressing an emotion – say of fear, sadness or surprise – the ability to read that emotion correctly is remarkably good. However, people vary in their ability to 'mind read' in this way. Individuals who are not adept at interpreting facial expressions find it more difficult to be empathic and as a result they are often less skilled at social relationships.

Emotions and Social Relationships

Awareness of other people's states of mind *vis-à-vis* the self and the ability to see the world from their point of view certainly facilitates the smooth running of social life, but it also has the power to generate some of our strongest feelings, both positive and negative. It therefore seems likely that there is some profound evolutionary significance in the co-existence of strong emotional states, group living, and our ability to be empathic and develop social cognition, that is imagine how things look from another person's point of view. As Oatley and Jenkins (1996: 91) recognize, the 'complex emotions of affection, gratitude, sympathy, empathy, compassion, provide the most important social glue'.

As we have seen, emotions give meaning to social life. They saturate what we say and do. A smile suggests warmth, acceptance, co-operation, affirmation and relaxation. A furrowed brow might indicate anxiety and doubt. The emotional tone of our dealings with one another is what gives relationships a certain kind of value and significance. Most of our strongest feelings are experienced in relationships. Failure to behave well in the group leads to feelings of shame. We avert our gaze, look down, drop our shoulders. Shame encourages conformity. Kindness from another makes us feel grateful. Someone who shares food or helps us with a task creates an emotional climate of co-operative bonhomie, so important if group living is to be successful. Gratitude promotes co-operation. Both shame and gratitude require us to evaluate our behaviour as we see it from the other's perspective.

Emotional talk appears to oil the wheels of everyday social life; it connects us to one another; it cements relationships. For example, Dunbar (1993) recorded hundreds of conversations between people in routine, daily situations. He found that what people talked about most was personal experience, relationships and social plans, with only a slight difference between the sexes (women 75%, men 65%). All talk and gossip about relationships has a very large emotional content, so that most mundane conversations contain a lot of reflection on and interpretation of one's own and other people's feeling states. Close relationships are also the place where we experience many of our most intense feelings, both positive and negative.

> Affectional bonds and subjective states of strong emotion tend to go together . . . Thus, many of the most intense of all emotions arise during the formation, the maintenance, the disruption, and the renewal of affectional bonds – which, for that reason, are sometimes called emotional bonds. In terms of subjective experience, the formation of a bond is described as falling in love, maintaining a bond as loving someone, and losing a partner as grieving over someone. (Bowlby 1979: 69).

Emotionally speaking, in most social relationships we are making constant adjustments. On the one hand we need to maintain good quality social interaction, while on the other to ensure our own needs and position are not lost. To the extent that we are mindful of the other's views and needs and the value of their contribution we might talk of love and affection, care and protection. To the extent we try to maximise benefits to the self we might talk of power, status, aggression and control (Kemper 1990). These two emotional elements – status and affection – are present to a degree in most social relationships but they may not be in balance. For example, the pursuit of power, status and control without the moderating effects of empathy and care can be socially destructive. What we tend to look for in relationships is warmth and recognition, love and acceptance, status and affection.

> We constantly monitor our own and others' behaviour in an effort to find clear direction and strategy for future behaviour. We need to be able to read each other's behaviour in order to know what's in store a little further on in the encounter. We need to repair any damage we've done in the form of apologies or promises. Having sensitivity and insight in the search for these

clues allows us to perform difficult social 'operations' such as helping ourselves or someone else, to maintain or retrieve dignity through face-saving rituals. (Layder 2004: 26)

Thus, in all relationships, there is a constant tension between the need for (i) relatedness/involvement/connectedness/dependence, and (ii) the need for recognition, separation and autonomy. We constantly try to adjust our behaviour to keep them in balance – a skill which is a measure of our emotional intelligence. Keeping the balance between *intimacy* and *autonomy* helps us to feel in control. It is when either intimacy or autonomy become too dominant that the self and the conduct of relationships get into social difficulty.

Similarly, many of the great themes of social interaction are captured as we struggle between love and anger, collaboration and conflict. Love and anger are the poles between which so much of our lives swing; they are the stuff of poetry and prose, song and drama. We are enraptured by the passions. It is in their exploration that we find our own essential being, a recognition and finally an understanding our selves.

Defining Emotions

Having explored the origin and function of the emotions, it is time to consider some definitions. In their excellent book on emotions, Oatley and Jenkins (1996: 96; also see Oatley et al 2006) offer the following working definition of an emotion:

1. An emotion is usually caused by a person consciously or unconsciously evaluating an event as relevant to a concern (a goal) that is important; the emotion is felt as positive when a concern is advanced and negative when a concern is impeded.
2. The core of an emotion is readiness to act and the promoting of plans; an emotion gives priority for one or a few kinds of action to which it gives a sense of urgency – so it can interrupt, or compete with, alternative mental processes or action. Different types of readiness create different outline relationships with others.
3. An emotion is usually experienced as a distinctive type of mental state, sometimes accompanied or followed by bodily changes, expressions, actions.

This definition identifies the key elements of our emotional life. Things happen to us that we *appraise* in terms of how they are affecting us or likely to affect us (Frijda 1986). Emotions therefore have a pervasive quality that affects the way our bodies as well as our minds feel. Our appraisals therefore become much more than simple computations of the objective properties of the situation. Our emotions give a fast, highly individualistic, subjective wash to what we see and experience. You miss the last bus home and decide to walk. Your thoughts are savouring the good time you have just enjoyed with friends. Then suddenly, the street lights along the quiet short cut you have just taken go out. You hear footsteps behind you followed by the jeering voices of a group of drunks. Their intimidating behaviour is frightening. It sets your heart racing as your body begins to shake and you try to walk faster, senses hyper alert. Quiet thoughts about the pleasures of the evening are overwhelmed and snubbed out by feelings of panic. You abandon the planned short cut and head as quickly as possible to the relative safety of the brighter lights of the busier main road. So:

> . . . emotions are things that happen to us rather than things we will to occur. Although people set up situations to modulate their emotions all the time – going to the movies and amusement parks, having a tasty meal, consuming alcohol and other recreational drugs – in these situations, external events are simply arranged so that the stimuli that automatically trigger emotions are present. We have little control over our emotional reactions . . . While conscious control over emotions is weak, emotions flood into consciousness. This is so because the wiring of the brain at this point in our evolutionary history is such that the connections from the emotional systems to the cognitive systems are stronger than connections from the cognitive systems to the emotional systems. (LeDoux 1998: 19)

Appraisal theory is therefore based on the assumption that each emotion is telling us something about our current relationship with the physical and social environment, that each emotion serves a particular adaptational function in a particular circumstance. Our minds and our bodies, both consciously and unconsciously, are monitoring and appraising how we are doing in this social encounter or that physical pursuit. The appraisal gives rise to a feeling, either positive or negative, with an implicit message to carry on or change tack, approach or escape, appease or avoid. Emotions rapidly excite us into a state of physiological and psychological readiness to deal with our concerns. They help prioritize goals, purposes and actions.

Events are constantly presenting us with problems to be solved. Evolution has therefore 'equipped humans with mechanisms that facilitate this problem-solving' (Parkinson 2004: 109). Emotions and the responses they trigger provide partial preformulated solutions to the problems met. 'Appraisal', continues Parkinson (2004: 109), 'determines the nature of the problem, emotion provides a strategy for its solution'. Emotions give us a quick, rough-and-ready response and orientation that help steer us through the first moments of the situation. In this sense, almost all situations, objects, people and memories bring about a quick burst of emotional arousal in us, however slight or short lived. Emotions provide us with an immediate, evaluative feel for the situation in which we find ourselves. These feelings give us our first pointer on how to respond to this person or that event. In short, 'Emotions occur at the juncture of our inner concerns with the outer world; they are evaluations of events in terms of their importance for our concerns' (Oatley 2004: 43).

For much of the time, we make sense of daily life through the cognitive lens of past experience which has taught us how things work and what to expect, especially in the context of relationships. It is when these expectations are not met that we experience a jolt and with it a reactive emotion. A father never gives his son a hug when they part, so when he does, the young man feels a strange mix of surprise, pleasure and puzzlement. When a quiet, previously mild-mannered elderly woman suddenly shouts at the indignity of her treatment, the care worker is startled and not a little frightened.

Appraisals are rarely conscious. In fact, probably the majority of emotions are triggered by appraisals operating at an unconscious level. Often it is only after an emotion has been experienced, that more conscious reflection and appraisal takes place, if at all. How explicitly aware are we that our low mood in the evening is the half sensed result of a series of minor set-backs and stresses throughout the day? And once in an emotional state, a good deal of mental activity is then generated by that state. If someone has hurt you, say by having an affair with your partner, a great deal of mental energy will be consumed by feelings of jealousy, anger and revenge that might include much emotionally heated fantasy – smashing his car windows knowing that he has been driving out with her, cutting up his favourite shirts, verbally and physically attacking the other woman. But other mental activities can also run alongside these angry thoughts. A degree of reflection begins to take place. The incident that precipitated the event that caused the emotion is analysed: I guess I've taken him for granted; I have felt irritated by his casual approach to life; we have been having more silly disagreements lately. These preoccupations are the beginnings of trying to make sense of a painful event and planning how to cope. Slowly, new plans – more adaptive to the new situation – begin to emerge leading to a new equilibrium.

Reflexes, Emotion and Cognition

Emotions lie somewhere between reflex responses and reflective cognition, between instinctive behaviour and conscious thought. Reflex behaviours are the things we do *without prior learning.* We are simply programmed biologically to behave this or that way whenever we meet a certain stimulus. In evolutionary terms, they are the most ancient aspects of our behavioural make-up. They are primitive responses to the environment. They give all species an in-built behavioural repertoire so that as soon as individuals are born, they automatically behave in a certain way under particular environmental conditions. Infants suckle breasts, seek out caregivers whenever they feel uncertain, explore whenever they feel safe. Of course, instinctive, reflex behaviours can be shaped by experience. These become 'learned behaviours'. Learned behaviour is just that – behaviour that is elicited when we meet a familiar experience or stimulus that may be positive (producing an approach response) or negative (leading to an avoidance response). Previous experience of that stimulus has 'rewarded' or 'punished' that particular behaviour so we do more or less of it whenever we meet that stimulus in the future.

Cognition or reflective thought assesses information, including how we feel about the experience. It is a more sophisticated response than either a reflex behaviour or an emotional reaction. In evolutionary terms, it is a relatively late development. In neurological terms, thought is relatively slow and so it isn't as useful as emotion in situations that demand a fast response. So although thought evaluates the accuracy of information, in survival terms emotions have their place, half way between reflexes and reflective thought. For example, when a large dark shadow swims beneath me in the water, I feel instantly wary and frightened. In my fearful state, I am well on my way to escape the danger before I have even given it much thought. Or, a surprise encounter with someone to whom I feel close causes me sudden joy and before I know it I have given her a big hug. It is only after the immediate emotional reaction that reflection makes me realize that the dark object in the water was nothing more than a rock, or before I knew it I was in a joyous embrace with an old friend.

So, lying somewhere between primitive reflex responses and conscious cognitive processing (thought), are the emotions. They help us make rapid judgements in situations of uncertainty and imperfect knowledge. So:

> . . . emotions are not just a biological quirk. They are a solution to a general problem . . . we have many different motivations or goals, and . . . emotions set priorities among them . . . Emotions function to manage our multiple motives, switching attention from one concern to another when unforeseen events affecting these concerns occur in the world, in the body, or in the mind . . . Emotions . . . point to the fundamental problematics of action in a world that is imperfectly known, and can never be fully controlled. (Oatley and Jenkins 1996: 253)

Very simple, reflexive organisms have no need of emotions. Similarly, a being with a perfect mental model of their environment who could predict, anticipate and respond absolutely appropriately to the world, again, would have no need of emotions. 'Everything is known, everything is anticipated' (Oatley and Jenkins 1996: 257). Perfect cognition could do it all. In reality, human beings fall somewhere between a simple bundle of programmed reflexes and a state of perfect knowledge. It is in this psycho-behavioural middle ground that emotions play their part. They give us some fast acting way of appraising and reacting to important features of our physical and social environment.

Emotions have evolved through their adaptive value in dealing with fundamental life-tasks (Ekman 1992). Without them we should be socially adrift, isolated and incompetent. Many behavioural and mental health problems are in fact little more than social dysfunction born of a lack of emotional skill, intelligence, awareness or understanding.

Conclusion

Oatley, Keltner and Jenkins (2006) report that the study of emotions is currently a fast moving field and caution against operating with a definition of emotions that is too fixed and inflexible. Nevertheless, they confirm that emotions are complex responses to the challenges and opportunities that are important to the tasks of daily living and survival, particularly those that are social in character. Whenever life stops us in our tracks and we become immediately aroused – it is then that we have *a feeling* and it is then that we act, one way or another, for better or worse. Our emotional character is the product of a long evolutionary history, embedded in our genes and social nature. However, for a full appreciation of our affective make-up, we need to look at how emotions develop over the life course. We need to examine emotional development in the context of parent–child relationships, family life and the cultural context.

4
Emotional Development

Introduction

If children and ultimately adults are to become competent social players, they must learn to manage both their own and other people's emotions. This will include becoming emotionally sensitive, aware and reflective. It will require an understanding of what causes feeling and how feelings affect us and our behaviour. Emotion regulation involves the modulation and control of our feelings and impulses, especially intense ones. Many emotions act as an internal guidance system, telling us what is important or acceptable, appropriate or dangerous, beneficial or risky (Wolfe 1999: 43).

Those who find it difficult to recognize and regulate their emotions will get into social difficulty. Anger causes aggression, shame leads to avoidance, sadness plunges people into depression. Emotional dysregulation upsets our ability to function well and effectively. Good mental health is based on the ability to recognize and regulate emotions. The breakdown of emotional order and control leads to poor mental health. The inability to regulate strong feelings is a major risk factor in psychopathology. It is therefore important to consider how children develop emotional skill and understanding. If they are not helped to recognize and make sense of feelings in the self and others, they are at risk of developing anti-social behaviours and mental health problems.

Nature and nurture both play a part in emotional development. In the journey from birth to full maturity, temperament, relationships with parents, the influence of family, and peer friendships help shape our emotional make-up and the very idea of a social self. If all goes well, emotional intelligence emerges and with it social wellbeing.

Temperament

It is in the interaction between babies and their caregivers, particularly at times of emotional arousal, that children's emotional development takes place. Temperament, which has a large genetic component plays a part in the interaction between nature and nurture. We vary in terms of whether we are naturally sociable or reserved, optimistic or pessimistic, cheerful or dour, extrovert or introvert, placid or fractious. These traits affect the basic tone of our emotional lives. They also affect how others respond. For example, shy people might instinctively avoid new, unfamiliar situations, including social opportunities. Caspi and colleagues (1987) have found that boys who showed a lot of anger at age eight years continued to experience relatively high levels of frustration and anger into adulthood. The angry trait appeared to affect their life chances, including the increased likelihood of poor marital relationships and employment records.

Kagan (1994), a strong believer in the fundamental influence that inherited temperamental traits play in our life and its prospects, argues that people seem to vary in terms of whether they are constitutionally timid or bold, melancholy or up-beat, inhibited or disinhibited. These genetic and constitutional characteristics interact with the social environment that includes mothers, fathers and their caregiving.

The work of Kagan (1994) has shown that many elements of an individual's temperament have a base in biology. For example, shy children are easily aroused even by low levels of stimulation. The emotional centres of their brains (limbic system) are very reactive. As a result they behave in a relatively inhibited, timid way when they are confronted by unfamiliar situations or potentially highly stimulating challenges such as rock climbing or negotiating new social situations. Timid babies are hyper-sensitive, behaviourally inhibited and more anxious. They are likely to grow into more timorous adults. They will be less confident when dealing with new experiences (food, situations, people) and so might be inclined to avoid them. They often subject themselves to feelings of guilt and self-reproach. Lying beneath this temperamental trait is a natural physiological sensitivity to stress, even mild stress. Anxiety is readily experienced. As adults, these over-sensitive, easily aroused individuals are more likely to suffer stress-related difficulties and associated health problems.

The nervous systems of timid, inhibited people are very easily aroused. However, if a timid baby is parented by a responsive and thoughtful carer, one who learns to graduate the child's exposure to novelty while ensuring that the child feels safe and able to cope with the increased arousal, these parents can help children build some resistance and levels of boldness. Hyper-sensitive, easily stimulated children therefore should not be overprotected but helped to feel they can control and deal with arousal. 'It appears that mothers who protect their highly reactive infants from frustration and anxiety in the hope of effecting a benevolent outcome seem to exacerbate the infant's uncertainty and produce the opposite effect' (Kagan 1994 pp 194–95). Babies need opportunities to learn how to manage and regulate their arousal, and so gain mastery over their own emotions and their regulation.

In contrast, extraverts require high levels of stimulation to experience significant arousal, hence their ready inclination to take part in thrill seeking sports and activities such as white-water rafting or bungee jumping, and to plunge into new social situations and opportunities. However, if the uninhibited child lives in a socially disadvantaged environment, opportunities for the expensive excitements of ski-jumping or parachuting will be limited. Thrills and stimulation might only be found in ways that are judged anti-social. Although racing stolen cars or playing chicken on a busy railway line might be sufficient to give an adrenalin-rush, they are far from acceptable pursuits to the community at large . 'Extraverts report more frequent and intense positive emotions than introverts, and high neuroticism individuals report more frequent and intense negative emotions than low-neuroticism individuals' (Rusting 2001: 375).

There is good evidence that an individual's emotional character, based on temperament, remains broadly consistent throughout childhood and on into adulthood. Short-tempered children are likely to become ill-tempered adults. Shy children often grow up to be quiet and reserved (Caspi et al 1987, 1988). These temperamental traits also predict some aspects of how people fare in life. Ill-tempered individuals are at risk of feeling dissatisfied in their relationships and experience higher rates of divorce. Shy boys become shy men who tend to marry later. Temperament and personality therefore appear to remain relatively stable over time. We tend to behave in characteristic and recognizable ways in similar situations. However, there is also strong evidence that relationships have a major influence on shaping how the individual experiences and self-manages these temperamental traits.

The Parent–Child Relationship

Although babies are born as emotional beings, at birth an infant's feeling states tend to be global and relatively undifferentiated. At any one time, the major emotions of fear, anger and contentment are experienced as immediate, total and all consuming. Babies can only communicate their anger and distress behaviourally. They cry and writhe. When they learn to crawl and walk, they can decrease some of their frustrations by making their own way towards their wants and desires. And with language, children begin to talk about their feelings rather than simply enact them with characteristic high intensity displays of behaviour. With maturation, therefore, children increase their ability to control the way they deal with and express their arousal.

Although babies are generally unable to regulate their own arousal, they do have a number of in-built, albeit basic coping strategies. For example, they can regulate emotional distress by turning their heads away from aversive stimuli in a form of gaze aversion. But most of the time, babies need help when they feel dysregulated, anxious and upset. Without help, very young children will continue to feel distressed until they exhaust themselves. They experience fear when they hear a loud noise. They feel angry when the breast is prematurely removed. The infant's day is made up of waves of these relatively unsubtle but strong emotional states. And because each emotion leads to very pronounced behaviours and facial expressions, each one helps babies powerfully to communicate their needs to those around them. Crying indicates distress caused by hunger or tiredness, alarm or pain. The cry of human infants can be extremely loud. For parents, the noise is certainly very compelling. Mothers and fathers in particular find their baby's cry very difficult to ignore. They are drawn to do something about it, that is they attempt to understand what is the matter and meet the need.

So, on their own, babies find it difficult to regulate their own arousal. What they need at times of distress is a comforting, containing, regulating relationship with another. If babies are to develop the ability to regulate their own emotions, their relationship with their primary caregivers is likely to be key. The sensitivity and comforting responses of the caregiver help infants manage and contain their upset. Sensitive parents are able to emotionally attune to their baby's experience and perspective. They acknowledge and understand that baby's have no choice but to communicate behaviourally, whether through crying or physical distress. Psychologically minded parents know not to take the crying and distress personally (Holmes 2006: 45).

Distress activates children's attachment system, the goal of which is to regain proximity to the caregiver. When contact has been achieved, the caregiver helps the child regulate her arousal using a variety of soothing and containing responses. This indicates to the baby that although her distress may feel all consuming, it is in fact manageable, it can be contained. Most of the senses are used by the caregiver to help the baby recover a sense of wellbeing. Touch, talk, singing, eye contact, cuddles, kisses, and nuzzles are used by parents and babies to communicate, to comfort, to connect, to calm. The mother's voice is slow, relaxed, rhythmical, quiet, gentle and soothing. The face expresses love and understanding. The infant's body is gently stroked and rocked. These soothing responses help comfort and calm the baby. All of this verbal, visual and tactile regulation typically accompanies the practical tasks of preparing a feed, having a bath, changing a nappy. Caregivers who can soothe and regulate, contain and manage arousal help their infants develop the capacity to 'mentalize', that is, make sense of their own and other people's emotional and mental states.

It might be noted that for most mammals, including humans, touch and physical contact is one of the most primitive and effective ways of regulating physiological and emotional arousal. Massage is a good way to help both adults and babies relax and relieve stress. Touch is at its most frequent and intense when we soothe babies (and when adults are in love). A number of relaxing, mildly sedating neurochemicals (natural opiates) including oxytocin, vasopressin and endorphins are released in the brain when we are caressed by another and whenever we experience the intimacy of a close relationship.

Co-regulation of affect between parent and child is important if maturing infants are to develop emotional intelligence and social competence. This sends a strong message to the baby that feelings can be understood, handled and contained. Both emotional regulation and self-organization emerge out of our relationship with others, particular with our caregivers and family. Moreover, as emotions give value ('valence') to experience and so help the brain organize its functioning, the regulation of emotions might be said to lie at the heart of self-organization (Siegel 1999: 278). This is why carers who are not good at reading their baby's emotional cues are in danger of compromising their child's healthy psychosocial development.

Smiling does occur in very young babies, but it is only by the age of three or four months that it seems linked to pleasurable experiences such as play and attention. Babies appear to get a great deal of pleasure from being able to control themselves and their environment. An infant will shake a rattle, make a predictable sound, and then laugh, before repeating the action. A four month old infant will locate and recognize his mother's voice and face, then smile. This indicates to the mother that she matters. Smiling babies are very attractive to adults. The smile is a positive, affirming emotional response, and it invariably draws the mother to interact affectionately with her infant, leading to further positive interaction.

During the first year of life, babies also begin to learn that other emotional expressions have communicative value. Anger suggests frustration, annoyance and dissatisfaction with what is happening, the implication being that the parent should do something about the disliked or disturbed state of affairs. A ball rolls out of reach; the mother leaves the room; food is withdrawn. In other words, emotions are not just expressions of internal states, they are increasingly directed at key caregiving individuals. And by the time babies reach the end of their first year of life, they are also monitoring their parent's emotional reactions. A frightened look from a father causes a child to hesitate before picking up a sharp knife carelessly left on the table. A smiling mother encourages her toddler not to be afraid and to join her paddling at the water's edge.

During the second year of life, children become increasingly interested in other people's emotional states, particularly distressed states. Many will attempt to give comfort, typically giving the other person something that the child would find comforting such as a favourite toy. There is clearly a prototype empathy occurring but it lacks the full features of an empathic response in which the other's view and needs are recognized and appreciated. However, by the age of three years, most children are beginning to understand that other people have an inner world of their own made up of thoughts and feelings. So when a young pre-school child sees another child hurt and crying, they are most likely to fetch that child's mother or father. The achievement of empathy is the basis of relationships and co-operation. It underpins socially skilled behaviour.

These early parent–infant interactions form the beginnings of a relationship, one in which the baby's arousal can be recognized and regulated, understood and managed. In effect, carers help shape their infants' early coping strategies. Repeated exposure to these regulating relationships help children begin to make sense of their arousal and what triggers and regulates it. Cognitive understanding also adds to the child's ability to achieve emotional regulation. Gradually, the young child realises that feelings can be thought about. In these ways, the child begins to rely less on the regulatory role of the caregiver. The toddler becomes increasingly emotionally self-controlled. However, the need to relate to other people at times of emotional stress never goes away. The emotional availability of other people and the desire for social support remain important whenever we feel hurt or sad, anxious or upset.

Learning to Recognize Emotions in Self and Others

One of the remarkable things very young babies appear able to do is recognize and discriminate between different emotional expressions on other people's faces and in their voices. They can also mimic some elements of the other's facial expression implying some in-built genetic ability to recognize and unconsciously copy expressed emotional states in other people (Field et al 1982; Haviland and Lelwicka 1987). This does not mean that the baby is actually recognizing the emotion as such, rather the infant is stimulated and reacts to certain features of the face that just happen to be involved in the expression of an emotion. Voice tone appears to be equally important in helping babies distinguish between emotions.

It is not absolutely certain whether negative emotions in young babies are simply experienced as undifferentiated distress or whether they can be recognized as discrete feelings of anger, fear, disgust or sadness that in turn are triggered by appropriate experiences (loss of a bottle, approach of a stranger, taste of something nasty, prolonged absence of carer). However, during the first year, interaction with carers begins to shape some of these innate states so that there is increasing correspondence between what elicits the feeling and a child's facial expression. Frightening events produce looks of fear. Surprising things elicit looks of surprise. And by toddlerhood not only do negative emotions become more differentiated, they are also expressed more intensely. For example, separation anxiety when the primary caregiver leaves a child is most frequent and intense between 15 and 18 months of age.

However, whether positive or negative, a baby's perceived emotional state prompts carers to react, responding affectionately when a smile occurs, or helping the infant deal with distress and discomfort. Either way, the child typically relates to the carer at times when he or she is emotionally aroused suggesting that the emotions are playing an important albeit complex role in the business of human relationships. It could also be the case that the baby's innate ability to imitate emotional expressions activates some existing, in-built neural response that generates the experience of the emotion being mimicked. In this way, the parent's display of an emotional state in response to the child's perceived mental condition is then mirrored by the infant who experiences something of the emotion being expressed. In this way, babies might be sharing affective states with the parent, an experience likely to help them in undertaking more sophisticated social interactions (Oatley and Jenkins 1996: 173).

With maturation, the young child begins to recognize that her own emotional behaviour affects others just as other people's emotions affect her. The subtle, rapid shift of affective states, in the self and others, helps children adjust their behaviour as they engage with others. Positive emotions increase pleasurable approach behaviour; negative emotions lead to withdrawal or trigger an aggressive approach. Positive feelings play a key role in interpersonal behaviour. They draw us closer together. Feeling happy inclines us to be more engaged and co-operative.

Emotional Attunement and Emotional Regulation

As we have seen, babies communicate their needs through vocalization, facial expressions and other behavioural displays of emotion. Babies appear programmed at birth to be particularly interested and stimulated by other people. In their early days, they are responsive to human voices, faces and eyes. The baby's gaze, in turn, stimulates the mother's gaze, and at this point of mutual eye contact, a potent, highly arousing line of communication and sharing of thoughts and feelings opens.

Infants seem to get a great deal of pleasure out of affecting and being affected by the behaviour and emotional state of other people. In turn, most adults seem to interact instinctively with babies by accentuating those channels of communication to which babies are neurologically highly attuned, even at birth, particularly facial expressions and voice intonation. In fact, much of the content of these exaggerated vocal and facial expressions is emotional in nature. Schore (1994) describe this as 'affect synchrony'. We tend to talk with babies in ways that seem instinctively designed to share and explore the feelings that the relationship itself engenders. Interacting rhythmically with babies – singing, rocking, stroking – seems instinctive to most parents. A musical quality is heard in our voice. When we talk with babies ('motherese' or 'infant directed speech'), our voice pitch tends to rise, tonal range is accentuated. Our speech has a slow, sing-song, rhythmical quality to it. Our pauses are relatively long, and there are fewer syllables per phrase. Trevarthen and Aitkin (2001: 8) further note that infants also prefer approving rather than disapproving voice intonation. Babies experience feelings of containment, regulation and safety as carers gently stroke, massage or rhythmically rock them in order to calm, soothe and reassure. All of this psychological and social interest, responsivity and reciprocity shown by babies is referred to as 'primary' or 'purposeful intersubjectivity'.

> Researchers found that as early as 2 months, infants and mothers, while they were looking at and listening to each other, were mutually regulating one another's interests and feelings in intricate, rhythmic patterns, exchanging multimodal signals and imitations of vocal, facial, and gestural expressions . . . Mothers and fathers were behaving in an intensely sympathetic and highly expressive way that absorbed the attention of the infants and led to intricate, mutually regulated interchanges with turns of displaying and attending. The infant was thus proved to possess an active and immediately responsive conscious appreciation of the adult's communicative intentions. This is what was called *primary intersubjectivity* (Trevarthen and Aitkin 2001: 5).

It is the mother's (or father's) sensitive perception and acknowledgement of these emotional states that enables her to make sense of her baby's inner feelings. Sensitive and emotionally attuned parents are also very good at reflecting back what they perceive their child's emotional state to be. This is known as 'affect mirroring' (Fonagy et al 2002; also see Winnicott 1967 on maternal mirroring).

Affect mirroring describes how carers credit their infant with an emotional state which they believe is *congruent* with the child's behaviour (angry cry, look of disgust, surprised reaction, frightened yell). If a mother thinks her baby is looking sad because the infant can't find his teddy bear, she is likely to mimic the baby's sadness by exaggerating her own facial and vocal expression of 'mirrored' sadness. 'Oh dear, who is looking so sad? What a sad face! Have you lost your teddy? Oh dear. Come on, let's find it and make you happy again.' From the baby's point of view, this is a kind of 'psychofeedback' in which 'my carer shows me my feelings' (Gerhardt 2004: 25). The carer's 'big' facial expressions and tone of voice give back to the child an idea of what the child is probably feeling. Mirroring takes the infant's distressed psychological state and organizes it for her. There is a physical, facial, emotional synchrony between mother and child (Stern 1977). Parents attempt to let children know that they recognize and understand what *they* are feeling, and how their feelings are affecting their behaviour.

These mirrored, attuned emotional signals serve either to amplify or dampen the infant's affective state so that distress is decreased and pleasure, or at least contentment is recovered (Schore 2001). If arousal gets too high, carers seek to calm things down. Or if a mother has over-excited her baby, say by playing a too boisterous game, and the infant starts to get upset or distressed, sensitive caregivers will withdraw and slow down the interaction. In broad terms, parents aim to keep their children alert and engaged, but not too overwhelmed nor too passive and under-involved. Of course, if a child is sleepy or unwell, attuned parents recognize that this is a time to be quiet, comforting, protective and caring. It is certainly not a time for play or stimulation.

In these ways, the maturing child begins to develop an understanding of her own psychological make-up and how she works emotionally. We learn to recognize and regulate our own emotional condition because we had carers who recognized and regulated our arousal when we were young. To be understood by another promotes self-understanding. 'Feeling felt' conveys a sense of deep emotional connectedness between mother and child. This is a pleasurable, reassuring, confirming and psychologically constructive experience. Children begin to recognize, understand and reflect on their own and other people's mental states and how these affect behaviour. These sympathetic mirrored looks are also the ones that most of us tend put on when we are acknowledging a friend's pleasure, or a colleague's sadness and pain.

Sensitive, attuned parents give their young children the strong message that emotions happen but they need not overwhelm us. Feelings can be thought about and understood. They can be contained and managed. Emotions also tell us interesting and important things about how we are currently experiencing our relationship with the world, particularly the world of other people. All of this marks the beginning of emotional self-regulation.

> None of us is born with the capacity to regulate our own emotional reactions. A dyadic regulatory system evolves where the infant's signals of moment-to-moment changes in his state are understood and responded to by the caregiver, thereby achieving regulation. The infant learns that the arousal in the presence of the caregiver will not lead to disorganization beyond his coping capabilities. The caregiver will be there to reestablish equilibrium. (Fonagy et al 2002: 37)

Most interactions between parents and young children tend to be positive, with expressions of warmth and enjoyment. In addition, babies who are cared for by emotionally sensitive parents quickly learn to discriminate emotional expressions on the faces of other people, typically in the sequence happiness first, then sadness, followed by anger and surprise. Emotional understanding and interpersonal awareness also develop as carers and babies interact and play for pleasure, companionship and stimulation. Story telling and verbal explanations of psychologically complex situations also help children to see the links between thoughts and feelings, emotional cause and effect.

Naming and Sharing Emotional States

Throughout their second year of life, with the help of their parents, children refer more and more to their own and other people's internal affective states. Parents begin to talk about thoughts and feelings much more frequently. Emotions are given names. Explanations are given about how feelings affect us, what causes them, and how they function. Children who develop high levels of emotional understanding tend to have mothers who are particularly expressive of emotions. Parents who relate with young children using relatively high levels of positive emotions have children who are more socially competent, have fewer externalizing problems, and who have a belief that with effort they can have an impact on their environment, particularly their social environment. Talk and discussion about negative feeling states is particularly effective in helping children recognize and understand the nature of their own and other people's emotions.

Families who acknowledge, enquire and talk about and reflect on feelings, families who are optimally and appropriately emotionally expressive, tend to have emotionally aware and socially competent children (Dunn et al 1991, Brown and Dunn 1996). These early signs of emotional intelligence also predict good relationships with peers. Socially skilled children are good at interpreting the emotions of their friends. This translates into successful entry into school life. In contrast, children who suffer poor emotional intelligence and are not good at regulating their emotions experience social problems at school. They are at increased risk of feeling isolated and sad (Fine et al 2003).

Children seem to be natural psychologists. Once they have acquired language, they constantly enquire about the reason why of things, particularly why other people are behaving the way they do. Much of children's talk is about how they feel. They ask questions about other people internal states, motivations and feelings: 'Why daddy cross? Why Emma sad? What is mummy laughing about?' These questions about behaviour invite a psychological answer. In order to understand other people's behaviour we need to know what is going on inside their heads. Behaviour is not random, it is not arbitrary. Behind it, people have motives, feelings, plans. Children begin to understand this. In order to make sense of the social world, they need to develop psychological understanding. In answering their children's questions, reflective parents give psychologically based replies. 'Daddy is cross because the car won't start.' 'Emma is crying because she is sad that her hamster has died.' 'Mummy is laughing because she's been given a nice present and that's made her very happy.'

On the whole, parents who convey a sympathetic concern for and understanding of their child's feeling states, particularly negative feelings, but who don't necessarily accede to the child's every want and wish or show support for less prosocial behaviours, these 'good-enough' parents with medium levels of responsiveness tend to have more socially competent children (Roberts and Strayer 1987). They appear to help their children deal realistically and flexibly with the complexities of social relationships including life's injustices. In turn, children of such parents are less stressed and more fluent in social situations.

These early explorations of emotional and social intelligence help the maturing child develop the 'ability to interpret others' behaviour in terms of mental states (thoughts, intentions, desires and beliefs), to interact both in complex social groups and in close relationships, to empathise with others' states of mind, and to predict how others will feel, think, and act' (Baron-Cohen et al 2000: 355). In essence, emotionally intelligent adults engage with young children as psychological partners. They credit infants and toddlers with minds, and that these minds are recognized, valued and worth knowing (Fonagy 2000). Reflective carers and parents constantly explain what is going on to young children in terms of the psychology of the situation, that all behaviour has a psychological underpinning, and that if other people are to make sense, then we need to consider them as thinking and feeling and motivated beings. If we are to understand others, we need to understand their interior life. Behaviour on its own is hard to fathom. Without consciously realizing it, parents train their children to be psychologists, astute observers and interpreters of the social and emotional scene. Emotional intelligence makes social life possible.

Children who can begin to think about and manage their own and other people's emotions are likely to handle themselves well in ever more demanding social situations. They get on well with their peers. Having friends and playing with your peers gives you further valuable social experience. Children who enjoy positive peer relationships learn even more about the importance of emotions and how they might be managed in the rough and tumble of the playground, the birthday party, the classroom. Emotionally literate children are the ones who help resolve conflict. They look for social solutions. They are less likely to resort to anger and aggression, avoidance and withdrawal. Pre-school children who do not respond prosocially to peers or who are not good at distinguishing between basic emotions such as happy and sad tend to be at risk for peer difficulties (Denham et al 1990). Popular children are more adept in understanding emotional situations; more prosocial; more empathic, constructive and flexible in sorting out emotionally-based interpersonal problems. They show better than average abilities to share, negotiate and develop co-operative play. These skills mean that they are likely to have friends and keep them.

In general, as people get older they tend to be more complex and differentiated in their emotional lives. They also place more value on emotion, processing emotional information more deeply. It is often surprisingly difficult for us to make sense of our emotions and feelings as they occur hence the value of talking about them and our fascination in seeing them played out and explored in drama, novels, tabloid press gossip columns, soap operas, and the cinema. In listening to other people's emotional experiences we gain understanding, empathy, emotional intelligence, social skill, and ultimately compassion. And those who are willing to listen empathically to another's hurt and stress bring comfort and reduce pain. Expressing and sharing positive feelings increases rapport and helps develop affiliative bonds. Self-disclosure about how we are feeling seems to be an integral part of achieving and maintaining intimacy. Those who are more reticent and tend to suppress emotional information and expression are less likely to achieve rapport or develop warm friendships and more likely to feel socially isolated and even self-alienated.

Adults who are able to describe their emotions in finer details and with greater discrimination rather than in broad, global terms tend to be much better at regulating their emotions (Feldman Barrett and Gross 2001). So, rather than simply describe oneself as feeling 'bad' or 'stressed out', much better to say that you are feeling a bit anxious and depressed, grumpy and maybe even rather cross as this predicts an increased ability to regulate emotional states. Individuals able to

discriminate in this fashion appear to have greater emotional awareness and therefore better information about what is happening and
how best to handle it. Regulation is even better if the individual can
begin to think about and identify the cause of each emotion: 'I'm
anxious because I'm being observed having contact with my children
this weekend, stressed-out because I haven't yet got round to sorting
out beds for the children if and when they are allowed to visit me at
home, depressed because my solicitor isn't optimistic about me
getting custody, and, grumpy and very cross because my ex-wife is
still telling lies about my behaviour towards her.'

Psychological Mindedness

Dennett (1987) believes that we try to make sense of each other in
terms of mental states. He also thinks that what goes on in other
people's minds in terms of thoughts, feelings, beliefs, and desires is
the key to understanding their actions and behaviour. If we are to
function effectively as social beings, we have to make sense of each
other at the psychological and emotional level. By the age of three or
four, most children develop 'a theory of mind', that is they recognize
that what people think, feel and believe is a good predictor of their
behaviour, even if what they believe is actually false.

For example, if Sally leaves her bar of chocolate on the kitchen
table and then goes out to play, the first place she will look for her
chocolate on her return is the table. However, in her absence her
mother has tidied the room and put the chocolate away in a
cupboard. On returning from the garden, Sally actually now has
a mistaken (false) belief that the chocolate is on the table; that is
where she left it, that is where she will expect to find it, and so that
is where she will first look. In order to predict Sally's behaviour, we
need to see the world from her point of view; we need to know that
even though she has a mistaken belief, nevertheless this belief will
predict what she will first do. When asked where Sally will first look
for her chocolate the moment she returns form the garden, most six
year olds get the answer right – on the table. Children younger than
three or four years of age tend to get the answer wrong. They hold a
literal view of the world. The chocolate is in the cupboard, so that is
where Sally will look. They lack a well developed 'theory of mind'.

This capacity for 'social understanding' based on the ability to see how things look and feel from someone else's perspective is the basis of empathy, relationship skills and moral behaviour. It also supports children's imagination and their ability to pretend and play. Having a good theory of mind helps people deal with the subtleties and complexities of social life. Indeed, without a theory of other minds an individual would be incapable of feeling many emotions, such as shame and embarrassment and the blushing that goes with them (Ramachandran 2003: 125; also see Crozier 2006 for a fascinating account of blushing and its relationship to embarrassment, shame and shyness).

Children and adults who suffer autism find it difficult to pass these theory of mind tests. They seem unable to appreciate that other people have mental states (thought, feelings, plans) that affect their beliefs and behaviour. As a result they find it difficult to see the world from the other person's point of view. Theirs is a very literal, behavioural world in which there is little understanding of the complexity of intersubjectivity and mentalization. Lacking this mental empathy and 'mind-mindedness', Baron-Cohen (1995) suggests they suffer 'mindblindness'. This is a major deficit that seriously impairs the ability to develop social cognition and emotional intelligence. Conducting relationships with skill and fluency is difficult:

> Imagine what your world would be like if you were aware of physical things but were blind to the existence of mental things. I mean, of course, blind to the things like thoughts, beliefs, knowledge, desires, and intentions, which for most of us self-evidently underlie behaviour. Stretch your imagination to consider what sense you could make of human action . . . if, as for a behaviourist, a mentalistic explanation was forever beyond your limits. (Baron-Cohen 1995: 1)

Meins (1997, 1999; also see Harris 1999: 317) argues that caregivers who are interested in what their children are thinking and feeling, and seek to share this understanding with their children are showing what she calls 'mind-mindedness'. Mind-minded parents are good at translating psychological experiences into an active, coherent dialogue with their children. This helps children link feelings and words. An emotionally attuned parent might ask a young child 'Are you worried that we'll be late for play group?' Or 'Are you feeling sad

because daddy's got to work away from home for a couple of days?'
Cozolino (2006: 232) reminds us that such questions guide children's
attention to their inner thoughts and feelings and how these affect
mind and body. Children are helped to understand that they have an
inner experience that is unique to them and different to those of
other people. Such mind-minded interactions facilitate emotional
understanding. Parents who focus on their children's subjective
experiences help them understand their own and other people's
psychological states. Understanding the origins, nature and effects of
emotions and their arousal helps children to manage their feelings in
a process of 'affect regulation'.

Emotional Development in Adversity

Babies and toddlers of carers who are insensitive and incurious about
their children's minds, thoughts and feelings – who lack mind-mindedness – do them a profound developmental disservice. As we have
seen, if children are to develop a theory of mind, empathy, social
cognition and emotional intelligence they need parents and families
who are fully engaged with them at the psychological level.

> If maternal care is not good enough, then the infant does not
> really come into existence, since there is no continuity of being;
> instead, the personality becomes built on the basis of reactions to
> environmental impingement. (Winnicott 1960: 54)

If your carers are neglectful or caught up with their own needs, anxieties and distress, their lack of interest in you and your mind starves
you of psychological information needed by your developing
psychosocial self in order for it to grow rich, complex and competent. Children find their minds in the minds of their carers. If you are
'out-of-mind' as far as parental interest and responsiveness are
concerned, then there is the danger that your absence in their mind
leaves you psychologically empty, incoherent, diffuse, incomplete.
Parents who are depressed or the victims of domestic violence, carers
who are trapped in hopeless poverty or addicted to drugs and alcohol, these parents risk neglecting their children at the physical,
psychosocial and emotional level. There is an air of helplessness
about these parents. They seem to lack both physical and mental

energy. They show little engagement with the world, including their children's needs, thoughts and feelings.

The evidence is strong that children who have suffered neglect and severe deprivation are at high risk of psychosocial impairment (Howe 2005). Their understanding of their own and other people's emotional character tends to be poor. Lacking emotional intelligence and psychological mindedness, neglected children are liable to a range of personal and social problems. Peer relationships are likely to be poor, depriving children of potentially useful social experience, thus depressing further their opportunities for more advanced psychosocial learning. Self-esteem might be low. Emotional intelligence is limited. Children react with confusion, distress or anger when they try to fathom and negotiate the challenges posed by peers and social relationships. These distressed reactions get them into trouble with parents and teachers. They are at increased risk of developing anti-social behaviours and mental health problems, particularly those associated with the 'internalizing disorders' such as anxiety and depression.

Some children suffer a different kind of adversity. Physical abuse, psychological maltreatment and emotional rejection witness a more active, but equally negative kind of caregiving. The child's needs and feelings are ignored by the parent. The caregiving is hostile, cold and critical. The child's dependence, even his vulnerability irritates and agitates the carer who deals with her upset by aggressively suppressing the cause of her uncomfortable arousal. The child might be contemptuously belittled. There is no sympathy for the tearful little girl who has fallen over and cut her knee: 'Stop crying. Don't be pathetic. Don't be a baby. Grow up and stop snivelling. It's only a scratch.' In more extreme cases, children might be slapped, punched and bruised. Some children are left in no doubt that their parents do not like them. 'I wish you'd never been born. You're a complete pain. I've got no time for you.' Emotional abuse and rejection are particularly hurtful. They leave deep psychological scars. Physically abused and psychologically maltreated children feel anger in the presence of dangerous caregivers but dare not express it lest it makes matters worse. There is fear of the hostile parent.

Abused and rejected children suffer heightened levels of a range of very negative emotions – fear, hurt, sadness, anger. However, it is their fate that although they experience feelings that are strongly dysregulating, they receive no parental help in their management or containment. It is therefore difficult for these children to understand or emotionally make sense of themselves or others, particularly when under stress. Feelings explode inside their heads. Maltreated children have few insights into the nature of their distress and arousal. In time, they begin to find the demands of most relationships stressful. Abused and rejected children typically behave very aggressively with their peers, with adults, and as they become bigger and stronger, even with the abusive and rejecting parents themselves. Lacking emotional intelligence and the regulating skills that such intelligence sponsors, these children grow into adults who are conflictual, aggressive, and anti-social.

However, we have to remember that deep down, these adults are in emotional pain. Not to feel loved or cared for by your parents – your attachment figures – is peculiarly hurtful. There is the nagging feeling that the self is unlovable, that to have been emotionally hurt and rejected by your parents might mean that you are unworthy and bad. The self can feel empty, worthless. Sometimes the individual feels attacked from within, a kind of self persecution from which there is no escape. Many adults who suffered childhood abuse and rejection try to escape and numb the psychological pain by turning to alcohol or drugs. Never having been helped to explore and feel comfortable with their own feelings, these adults avoid emotional intimacy. They defend against the upset that hides beneath their fragile shell of indifference by dismissing feelings, constantly presenting themselves as strong, emotionally hard, and contemptuous of intimacy, weakness and need.

Beeghly and Cicchetti (1994) found that children who had experienced severe neglect and abuse used significantly less 'internal state language', that is they talked less about their own thoughts, feelings and actions than non-maltreated toddlers. They were also less able to differentiate between feelings. For example, they were confused between their feelings of sadness, anger and fear. And on top of this, their range of feelings also appeared limited and rather blunted. One effect of these affective deficiencies is the inability of many maltreated children to regulate their own arousal or to differentiate, label and understand emotional expressions in other people.

Abused and neglected children show a poverty of responses and lack variability and flexibility when dealing with the routine demands and stresses of social relationships. There is now strong evidence that all forms of child abuse and neglect increase the risk of mental health and psychiatric problems. Whenever clinical and psychiatric populations are examined, there is an over-representation of people who have suffered maltreatment as children (Kaufman and Charney 2001).

The Emergence of the Self and the Social Emotions

Intimately involved in the ability to be socially competent is the very sense of self. Our sense of self only emerges in relation to other people. The self and self-understanding are created during interactions with others. Through countless interactions young children begin to develop an increasingly robust sense of an independent self, with a mind in which there are thoughts and feelings. But with the clear emergence and recognition of the self comes the potential for other emotional states including embarrassment. Whereas fear can be triggered from a very young age and occurs without a concept of self, shame and embarrassment seem to require a sense of an independent self performing inadequately, inappropriately and ineffectively in the company of other people.

Emotions are often most intense in the context of social relationships. In pre-school children, negative emotions in particular tend to receive a lot of thought and explanation, both by the children experiencing the emotion and other children watching its display. Negative emotions are important states to handle in social relationships which is why they probably demand so much mental work by both subjects, recipients and observers. As children become more aware of their own and other people's emotional states and how they affect behaviour and interaction, for good or ill, they also learn to control emotional expression. They may even try to mask feelings. Older children realize that showing disappointment on receipt of an inappropriate present from an aunt is not socially acceptable, so they feign pleasure and gratitude. They begin to recognize that other people are also living these complex emotional lives in which feelings can be hidden, feigned and dissembled.

Children's growing ability to 'mentalize' and to make sense of themselves and others as psychological and intentional beings provides them with high levels of resilience. They begin to see the world of people as fathomable. Other people's feelings and behaviours are not arbitrary and random. Behaviour happens for psychological reasons. The gradual appreciation of otherness, including the realisation that others hold a mental view of you, is also critical to the development of the psychological self, self-awareness, intentionality and emotional intelligence.

Social Sharing of Emotions

When our emotions are running high, we tend to seek the company and conversation of others. We have a drive to share our emotions, to explore them, to try and make sense of them as we talk about our feelings with family and friends (Rimé et al 1998). Whenever we have had a significant emotional experience, whether positive or negative, we tend to share it with other people, though shame and guilt are more likely to be kept to the self. We describe the event and the feelings it triggered, often in great deal. Close friends, family and intimates are the people with whom we are most likely to share emotions, although if the emotional event is a professional or work-related matter, colleagues will also be chosen. Typically, most of us tend to repeat the story to other people so that over the space of a few days or weeks the incident might be described many times over. The more intense the emotion, the more often it is shared and for a longer time (Rimé et al 1998). Why do we do this?

Conventional wisdom suggests that talking about significant emotional experiences is cathartic. By talking about emotionally charged experiences, we give vent to our feelings, and somehow discharge their potency and capacity to dysregulate. The emotional load is lightened. Indeed, when people are asked, most say that they found talking to a sympathetic listener about their feelings helpful and beneficial even though the emotional potency of the experience did not lessen (Zech et al 2004). But research findings spin this picture slightly differently.

Sharing emotions increases feeling socially supported by family, close friends and valued colleagues. It cements affiliative bonds and promotes social consensus and integration. This is particularly pronounced when the other shows empathy, interest, validation and understanding. If the emotion being described is particularly intense, words are sometimes not enough. In these cases, the sensitive or consoling listener might simply touch or hug or kiss their close friend depending on whether the emotion is one of upset, anxiety, sadness or sheer joy. Further benefit is derived when the other shares their own similar experience, adds new information, invites alternative ways to think about the emotional event or even gives advice. Emotional sharing helps clarify feelings and promotes self-understanding. There is also evidence that those who are more prepared to be open and use self-disclosure in close and intimate relationships are more liked than those who are more reticent and withholding.

So, sharing feelings with others both maintains and helps establish close relationships. However, the choice of confidant depends on age and situation. Children share most of their important emotions with their parents, but as they get older, friends become increasingly important, especially in adolescence. Adults are most likely to share their feelings with romantic partners, although friends, particularly female friends and work-colleagues remain important. People often say they feel closer after an emotion has been shared.

It therefore appears that although sharing emotions does not of itself lessen the immediate strength of the emotion's intensity, it does increase people's sense of social belonging and reduces feelings of isolation and confusion. Giving voice to feelings in relationship with an empathic other helps make sense of the emotion, gives meaning to the experience, and so helps the individual feel more in control.

More generally, co-operative behaviour has proved key to the evolutionary success of human beings. Social skills and the ability to develop co-operative behaviour are developed in children's play. Play can be of the imaginative kind between two young friends. Small groups might playfully construct a bridge of logs across a small brook. Or larger groups gather to play a game of football or netball in which rules have to be followed if the game is going to work. Children, and indeed adults, derive a great deal of fun and happiness getting involved in games and working together constructively. It is no accident that we often say that we pursue these activities for 'pleasure'. If we derive intense pleasure from either the activity or the relationships that facilitate it, we say we 'love' playing that game or we are great friends with these people. The loss of the activity or the people is disappointing and leads to feelings of sadness.

We seek to regulate our emotions as we move in and out of different situations during the course of each day. Generally, though not always, we try to suppress anger knowing that its unbridled expression will be viewed negatively by others. If a colleague turns up late to an important meeting, we might attempt to control our feelings of anger and irritation. When a child first learns to ride a bike, parents react with exaggerated glee and praise. Or if an acquaintance wins a car as first prize, we are more likely to congratulate her on her good luck than express our envy which is perceived as a mean and unworthy emotion.

Fischer et al (2004: 188) quote Gross who says that emotion regulation refers to those processes by which 'individuals influence which emotions they have, when they have them, and how they experience and express these emotions'. Regulation might be achieved by be reappraising the situation or avoiding it or deliberately suppressing our reaction to it. But before we can do this, we first have to be able to be aware of and recognize our own emotional condition. This then allows us to monitor any discrepancy between the feeling that we have and the appropriateness of its expression.

Culture and Emotions

Other people and their opinions play an important part in the way we regulate our feelings. We take into account the likely reactions of others. We do not like to be seen as going against emotional norms. Our emotions and their expression are regulated with reference to our perceptions of what is culturally appropriate. Most of us feel extremely uncomfortable, even abnormal if we think we are being seen as behaving in an emotionally different or deviant way. Although we might generally be inclined towards being emotionally up-beat, nevertheless, if we think smiling would be 'bad form' in particular company under certain circumstances we are likely to suppress that emotion as part of our 'impression management'. Even though we have just accepted a new and exciting job, smiling gleefully at the funeral of a great aunt would be bad form. Our social experiences therefore construct a large part of our psychological interior. We begin to think and feel in ways that are culturally appropriate.

The need for adjustment of our emotions thus lies largely in the need to live the good social life. Being too frightened, or too angry, or too sad is a problem not so much for our biological system, but rather for our social system. It is not surprising therefore that appropriate emotion regulation is seen as a core ingredient of an emotionally intelligent person ... Individuals who do not respond emotionally in an adequate manner may survive physically, but will become social outcasts. (Fischer et al 2004: 188)

With this in mind, continue Fischer et al (2004), on the whole we are motivated to please and protect others rather than to hurt or offend them. But in our social interactions, we are also trying to influence and manage other people's views of, feelings about and behaviour towards us. However, the more self-conscious we become about such emotional matters, the more our reference point becomes the injunction to remain true and authentic to our feelings. Over the last few decades this has certainly become true in the West with its increasing emphasis on emotional sensitivity and emotional intelligence. In this we might detect a slight shift away from the social group as the perceived arbiter of emotional appropriateness to the self as the measure of emotional integrity and authenticity.

Anthropologists have long recognized that different cultures have different understandings of and give different values to certain feelings. Indeed, some feelings, common and important in one culture go unrecognized and without value in another. In the West, seen as an 'individualistic culture', the self is valued as independent, assertive and essentially separate from others. To be authentic is to remain honest and true to your own feelings and desires. The display of emotion is not only acceptable, but it is often regarded as healthy.

In the East, seen as a 'collectivistic or honour culture', the self is felt, experienced and valued much more in relationship with others. Interdependence with others is key, and for this to be threatened is the cause of anxiety and shame. The self is woven into the social fabric, and many strong feelings, either positive or negative, arise as the self relates supportively with or separately from the group. Emotions help mediate social relationships. Lutz (1988) believes that in these cultural cases, individuals experience emotions at the group level rather than individually. In other words, emotions arise in relationship with others. However, whether East or West, this is probably true of most of our strongest feelings. It is in relationship with others that we are most likely to experience sadness, anger or embarrassment.

> In collectivistic cultures, the norm to maintain harmony within one's ingroup should elicit the norm of suppressing those emotions that create tensions or distance between people, such as anger, contempt, annoyance, or pride. On the other hand, there is a norm to display emotions that show one's interdependence with others, such as shame, guilt, friendly feelings, or feelings of respect. In individualistic cultures, the opposite pattern can be found. Westerners are reluctant to show emotions, such as shame, that display their faults or weakness, and therefore place a taboo on these emotions. Emotions that emphasize one's independence, assertiveness, or uniqueness, on the other hand, are encouraged. (Fischer et al 2004: 193–4).

In spite of these cultural differences, all human beings have to negotiate the need to be both independent (in which one's actions are organized by one's own internal preferences, attributes and personality traits) and interdependent (in which one's actions are organized by roles, duties and social obligations). To a degree we all need to develop a sense of an independent psychological self. But we also have to feel connected to social groups if we are to survive (Kitayama et al 2004: 253–4). There is therefore a tension between dependence and interdependence, with the East leaning more towards interdependent answers and the West towards solutions based on the self being seen as primarily independent.

Conclusion

Emotional intelligence is born out of good quality, psychologically-minded relationships, and emotional intelligence allows us to enjoy and benefit from the company of others. Emotions and their understanding are refined and shaped throughout our early years as we relate with parents, family and friends. Throughout the life course, relationships continue to be where we experience many of our most intense feelings. We turn to others whenever we want to grapple with strong emotions. Relationships remain important in helping us regulate arousal and alter mood and outlook. Emotions are therefore typically recognized as a psychological experience, often cast in a social setting. However, emotions in particular and our psychological states in general are not some free-floating phenomena. They are the product of our brain and its workings. Indeed, the brain turns out to be the organ that links mind and body. If we are to have a full understanding of our emotional selves, we need to appreciate what is happening in the brain as we freeze with terror, feel overcome with love, or cringe with shame.

5
The Emotional Brain

Introduction

Over the last couple of decades, scientists have begun to understand some of the links between our brain's biological make-up and our psychological experience. Advances in ways we scan, image and monitor the brain's activities in real time have had a great impact on the neurological sciences. This has been particularly true of our understanding of the emotions. The title of this chapter is a straight steal from LeDoux's 1998 landmark text, *The Emotional Brain*. As the subtitle of his book suggests, LeDoux explores 'the mysterious underpinnings of emotional life'.

For many social workers, talking about the brain might come as something of a surprise. But as neuroscientists begin to make sense of the neurological basis of feeling, behaviour and mental health, the relevance to those who work with people in distress and difficulty becomes clearer. Those who cannot regulate their emotions will soon get into social difficulty, whether their dysregulated condition is based on inherited traits, organic problems, upbringing, illness or disease that affects the brain and its functioning. An interest in the brain and how it functions (and malfunctions) is rapidly beginning to inform the knowledge-base of all the people-oriented and relationship-based professions including clinical psychology, psychotherapy, counselling, nursing and medicine. It therefore seems timely to introduce the brain and its working to a social work audience. The science of the brain is fiercely complicated, but a brief overview should sensitize us to some of the biological processes that drive our emotional life and social behaviour.

The Complex Brain

We need to remind ourselves that the brain is an extraordinarily complex organ. It is made up of 100 billion neurons or nerve cells.

Each cell is connected with many other cells via dendrites and axons that meet the axons and dendrites of other cells. In reality, a small gap exists between the axon of one cell and the dendrite of another known as the 'synaptic gap'. Although electrical signals activate and move through each cell, this signal gets converted into a chemical messenger at the synaptic gap. The chemical messenger – or neurotransmitter – moves across the gap and triggers an electrical signal in the adjoining cell. There are many kinds of neurotransmitter and they play a major part in the way our brains work. If these neurotransmitters are out balance or upset by other chemicals that are introduced into the brain (alcohol, drugs, medicines), then we may experience changes in our mental processes, emotional states, moods and behaviour.

Any one cell may be connected to anything between 1,000 and 100,000 other cells. That is, each cell may have thousands of synapses. It will be apparent that the number of synapses, or neuronal connections, is astronomical. 100 billion cells each with thousands of synapses means that there are trillions of neurological connections present in the human brain, often arranging themselves in intricate webs generating systematic patterns of interaction. No wonder that trying to examine and understand the brain and how it works is such a challenge. Nevertheless, this shear complexity also begins to explain why the brain is capable of such wonderful and diverse tasks including managing and regulating the body and all its functions, including thoughts, feelings, perception, language and memory. It is also a powerful reminder that when any part of the brain is damaged or disturbed it is likely to have a profound affect on our behaviour and functioning. A brain injury might cause paralysis of the legs, disease might lead to loss of short term memory, a stroke could impair speech.

The Social Brain

The brain clearly controls, monitors and processes many aspects of both body and mind and many of its capacities are in-built and are present at birth. However, many of the brain's processing and interpreting functions are achieved during development, particularly in the early years. In order to cope with and adapt to environments of physical and social complexity, it makes more sense to tailor-make your understanding and responses to the particular characteristics of those environments in which you are going to have to function and survive. If your brain came fully programmed at birth, your behavioural repertoires and intellectual abilities would be rigid, invariant and extremely limited and limiting.

So the human brain, similar to the brains of many mammals, does much of its neurological 'hard-wiring' after birth. Much of the brain is therefore programmed to make sense of experience but it needs exposure to experience of which to make sense before it can make sense. This is true of so many of our potential capacities including sight and language.

For example, although our eyes receive and focus light signals which then stimulate the optic nerve, only when these visual stimuli are received at the back of the brain in an area known as the occipital lobe do we then 'see' what is out there. It is the brain that 'sees' not the eyes as such. But the brain has to learn to make sense of these visual inputs and it does this over the first few months and years of life. By the end of the 'learning to see' process, the brain manages to create a coherent picture of the external visual world having learned to process and integrate all the component bits of vision including contrast, colour, texture, perspective, movement and so on. During this process millions of neurons are being repeatedly stimulated, sending out dendrites and making synaptic connections with other neurons to create a highly complex neurological structure that processes incoming signals giving us our sense of sight and vision. The more frequently particular clusters of neurons are fired in response to certain visual inputs, the stronger the synaptic connections between those neurons. Thus, the hardest working neurons make the most effective connections.

If the brain is denied exposure to visual stimuli during this sensitive phase of development, not only do neurons in the visual cortex fail to 'fire', they also fail to connect with one another. In a process known as 'pruning', neurons that are not used and fail to make dense connections with other neurons die. These processes illustrate Hebb's famous principle that 'nerve cells that fire together wire together' and, neurologically speaking, we have 'to use it or lose it' (Hebb 1949). In short, the brain is a self-organizing developmental structure that constructs itself in the light of experience to make sense of that experience in a process known as 'structural neuroplasticity'. In this way, individuals and their brains become adapted to the particular environment (physical, language, emotional, interpersonal, cultural) in which they find themselves. This is both developmentally exquisite and a neat biological trick.

This basic thesis has been well researched in many species including humans. Indeed, for their groundbreaking work on how the brains of cats learn to see, Hubel and Wiesel (1962) received the Nobel prize. However, in reality matters are more complicated even than this. Areas of the brain that are not used to process and interpret one sense, such as vision, may in part be taken over by other intact senses, such as touch or sound as might be the case for children born blind. The remaining senses might become more acute as they colonize other areas of the brain giving that sense more neurological 'computing' power.

More recent work has extended our understanding of neurological development to examine how we begin to process, recognize and interpret emotions and other social phenomena. Indeed, so much of what we need in order to become competent human beings requires that large parts of the brain become linked and integrated to make sense of socio-emotional experience. Many neuroscientists go so far as to say that the relatively large size of the human brain is because the challenge of processing and interpreting complex interpersonal experience is such a big task.

Similar to the process of learning to see, we need exposure to good quality social and emotional information in order to make sense of ourselves and other people as complex emotional, psychosocial beings. Our 'social brain' is constructed in relationship with others in order to make sense of social interaction. In these ways, our complex, experience-dependent brains allow us to adapt to the intricacies and elaborate demands of our social environment.

To accomplish the goal of building a social brain, evolution has selected for 'bonding, attachment and caretaking to provide the necessary scaffolding for the prolonged extrauterine development. This "socialization" of the brain laid the foundation for increasingly sophisticated forms of communication, the emergence of language, and the birth of culture' (Cozolino 2006: 295). In this sense, the 'baby is an interactive project not a self-powered one. The baby human organism has various systems ready to go, but many more that are

incomplete and will only develop in response to other human input.'
(Gerhardt 2004: 18).

The downside of our experience-dependent brain, as with vision, is that if we are not exposed to good quality socio-emotional experience, the brain will either develop in the light of the social and emotional experience to which it has been exposed, no matter how disturbed, or, in the case of extreme emotional neglect and deprivation, fail to develop the relevant neurological architecture even to begin to handle social and emotional experience in anything like a competent fashion. Children who have been raised from very young ages for very many years in severely socially deprived institutional environments suffer severe neurological and psychosocial impairments. These set-backs adversely affect deprived children's ability to develop intersubjectivity, emotional intelligence and social skills. This is how Cozolino (2006) summarizes matters:

> The fact that the brain is such a highly specialized organ of adaptation is both good and bad news. The good news is that if unexpected challenges emerge, our brains have a greater chance to adapt and survive. When good-enough parenting combines with good-enough genetic programming, our brains are shaped in ways that benefit us throughout life. And the bad news? We are just as capable of adapting to *unhealthy* environments and *pathological* caretakers. The resulting adaptations may help us survive a traumatic childhood but impede healthy development later in life. Our parents are the primary environment to which our young brain adapts, and their unconscious minds are our first reality. Because the first few years of life are a period of exuberant brain development, early experience has a disproportionate impact on the development of neural systems. In this way, early negative interpersonal experiences become a primary source of the symptoms for which people seek relief in psychotherapy. (Cozolino 2006: 6–7, emphasis original)

The Evolutionary Origins and Organization of the Brain

The more scientists examine the brain, the more complicated and interconnected its structures appear to be. However, according to MacLean (1990), the modern human brain is made up of three basic parts: the brainstem, the limbic system, and the cortex. This probably oversimplifies matters, but the divisions help us gain a basic idea of how and why the brain's architecture is the way it is.

Brainstem

The most basic and ancient part of the brain is known as the *brainstem*. It lies deep in the brain at the base of the skull surrounding the top of the spinal cord. It controls all those functions of which we are unaware but which need to take place if we are to stay alive. Amongst many things, these functions include regulating body temperature, breathing, movement, digestion and metabolism. The brainstem also provides us with a number of basic 'behavioural scripts' which also lie outside consciousness. These scripts give pattern and shape to the way we proceed through each day. We wake, we eat, we defecate, we manage our 'territory', we interact, we settle and go to sleep. This primitive part of our brain is also involved in sexual feelings and behaviour. It is concerned with survival in the sense of staying safe which might include fighting off danger.

As such, the brainstem does not 'think'. It operates as a set of pre-programmed monitors and regulators. Because the brains of some creatures such as reptiles are made up mainly of brainstem and only a little cerebral cortex, this part of the brain is sometimes known as the 'reptilian brain'. Damage to this region can affect our ability to be purposeful and organize our day and its rhythms. For example, individuals who suffer the hereditary disease Huntingdon's chorea will simply sit and do nothing unless encouraged to do otherwise. More serious injury to the brainstem means death as it controls so many of our basic bodily functions.

Limbic system

The *limbic system* is sometimes known as the emotional centre of the brain. This is true in so far as the limbic system does play a major part in our experience of feeling, but other regions of the brain are also involved in emotional experience. Nevertheless, the brain induces emotions from only certain parts of the brain, many of them located beneath the cerebral cortex including the brain stem, hypothalamus, the anterior cingulated region, basal forebrain, and amygdala

(Damasio 1999: 61). Different emotions are likely to involve different parts of the brain. In other words, each emotion involves the activation of a distinct pattern of neurological sites. Specific damage to any one or more of these areas, caused by disease or accident, will adversely affect our ability to perceive or experience particular emotions.

In broad terms, the limbic system lies in the centre of the brain beneath the cortex, surrounding and sitting on top of the brain stem in a ring-like fashion, hence the name 'limbic' from the Latin for border, rim or edge. As we have noted, strictly speaking, the limbic system is not a clearly defined region of the brain, but for our purposes the term acts as a useful shorthand for those regions that do seem to be especially involved in processing emotional stimuli and our responses to them. Interestingly, the limbic system is also where some of the neural pathways associated with smell terminate. This is why some smells seem to have the power to call up emotion laden-memories. A particular scent or perfume, the smell of a school classroom or new mown grass might suddenly conjure long forgotten memories and feelings.

In evolutionary terms, the emergence and growth of the limbic system seems to be associated with species that are social, group living, look after their young, form attachment bonds, and play, especially when young. Species that communicate also seem to have well developed limbic systems. This gives us a strong clue about the nature of emotions and why human beings might have them in such rich abundance. The common thread through all the above activities is social interaction. It looks as if species that are good at interpersonal, co-operative behaviour need to experience emotions and have feelings. Emotions seem to play a key part in generating information about how we are doing as we interact and relate with others.

As we saw in Chapter Four, we have faces and vocalization capacities that are able to express a wide variety of emotions. Our extremely mobile faces with their complex musculature allow us to communicate a whole range of feelings including affection, love, fear, sadness, surprise, disgust, embarrassment, and anger.

So, there seems to be some deep linkage between our social nature and the fact we have social emotions, and that these emotions can be communicated. Most fish, amphibians and reptiles, in contrast, have expressionless faces and rarely vocalize. Other than during mating, reptiles, amphibians and fish do not behave socially although they do experience some of the basic emotions of survival such as fear. We might deduce, therefore, that complex emotions somehow oil the social wheels, allowing us to function more effectively as a group-living, co-operative species. Emotions seem to add an extra dimension to our experience and give us evolutionary advantages. However, viewing emotions in this way also points to the potential problems that an individual might suffer should he or she experience difficulties recognizing, understanding, interpreting, regulating or communicating his or her feelings. Emotional dysfunction translates into relationship difficulties which become social problems, and social problems increase the risk of personal distress, mental health difficulties, and behavioural incompetence.

A small, but important part of the limbic system is the *amygdala,* a name derived from the Greek for almond because of its shape and size. It receives sensory inputs from many senses including the eyes and ears. Sensory information can go directly to the amygdala, bypassing the cortex. In other words, we can experience a strong feeling *before* we become aware of it and have time consciously to think about it. From an evolutionary point of view this is important. Information that is handled by the conscious, thinking part of the brain – the cortex – is processed relatively slowly. If there is a threat to the individual, any neurological processing that is slow delays survival responses and so increases the danger. By going direct to the amygdala, we experience an immediate sense of fear that triggers an escape response, even before we have had time to think. Our hearts pound and we find ourselves running away, or we shiver, freeze and become ultra alert and aware. As we discussed in Chapter Three, emotions are therefore quick appraisal, fast response experiences that often happen before we have time to reflect and take stock. Anger, fear, elation, embarrassment or surprise burst into our heads and bodies as we attack, run away, scream with joy, blush and look down, or stare in transfixed fascination at the unexpected or unusual.

Thus, upon receipt of a sensory input, the amygdala appraises the experience and gives it an immediate emotional value or 'valence' which leads to a fast action response. The amygdala is therefore a site of primary appraisal, where events are automatically evaluated in relation to the individual's goals and concerns (Oatley et al 2006: 148). Appraisals that evaluate a stimulus as positive generally lead to approach responses, while those assessed as negative cause us to avoid and turn away from the person, object or situation. Emotions are the conscious experience of these largely unconscious evaluations.

The work of LeDoux (1998) notes that the amygdala is particularly important in the appraisal of fear. Fear, of course, is one of our most basic, powerful, important, and deeply remembered emotions. It is to do with our very survival, our very existence. When we are frightened the whole of our mind and body reacts as we are flooded with feelings of alarm and danger. Blood drains from the skin and is diverted to the long muscles as our bodies go into flight and escape mode. We therefore shiver and feel cold. Our hearts pound faster as blood carrying oxygen and energy is pumped to the arms and legs to help as run, or if necessary fight and defend ourselves.

For the very young and dependent, feelings of fear and distress are easily activated. When you are small and very vulnerable, danger is ever present and survival is precarious. Secure infants enjoy a protective, emotionally regulating relationship with their caregivers and so learn to manage anxiety. Abused and neglected, abandoned and rejected children may not have such protective, containing experiences with their attachment figures. Matters are made even worse when the source of danger or abandonment is the parent himself or herself. The person who should be a safe, protective haven at times of danger turns out to be the danger. This can be a particularly traumatic experience for small children. Such trauma can overwhelm the young brain. In these cases, the amygdala is massively aroused and retains traumatic memories that lie outside language (the young brain not yet having developed its language processing abilities).

Traumatic experiences in the first two years or so of life profoundly affect the 'deeper' structures of the brain that are responsible for regulating our bodies, senses and emotions, particularly when we are under stress. Literally, many traumatic experiences, especially early ones, cannot be described or put into words. They are simply experienced as an overwhelming feeling of fear and danger.

Severely compromised attachment histories, explains Schore (2001a: 16), 'are . . . associated with brain organizations that are inefficient in regulating affective states and coping with stress, and therefore engender maladaptive infant mental health'. Perry and Pollard (1998) are clear that early life maltreatment adversely alters the organization, structure and density of the emotional processing parts of the brain, permanently robbing children of a normal psychosocial development (De Bellis 2001: 552).

Fonagy (2001: xv) develops this line of thinking, adding that 'the average human mind is simply not equipped to assimilate or protect itself from environmental assaults beyond a certain intensity'. By far the most intolerable of such assaults are those that occur in relationship with the very people who are biologically earmarked to protect you, your caregivers. The brains of seriously abused and neglected children have an impaired capacity to regulate impulse and emotions. 'Both lack of critical nurturing experiences and excessive exposure to traumatic violence will alter the developing central nervous system, predisposing to a more impulsive, reactive, and violent individual' (Perry 1997: 131). This will have implications in terms of later social behaviour.

The more traumatic, hostile and rejecting the caregiving, the more the brain's healthy development is compromised. Severe sexual abuse, psychological maltreatment, emotional abuse, relational trauma, rejection, and emotional unresponsiveness impair the developing brain's 'hard-wiring' (Joseph 1999, Schore 2001b, Balbernie 2001). In particular, the traumatised child's and adult's ability to process and regulate emotional arousal is severely disturbed. The risk of mental health problems, relationship difficulties and social problems is high amongst those who carry unresolved issues of loss, abuse and trauma into adulthood. Little surprise therefore that so many of those involved in domestic violence, depression, substance abuse, child maltreatment, and violent offending behaviour have had sad, distressed and painful childhoods.

We have seen that because the amygdala is connected directly to our senses, it creates strong and powerful feelings. Not surprisingly, therefore, it is also implicated in certain kinds of learning and memory. Many key behaviours (whether of approach or avoidance) are learned when our emotions are running high. And some of our most vivid and evocative memories are associated with emotionally charged events. The more frightening or thrilling or extraordinary the situation, the more the amygdala is aroused and the more likely it is that situations of that kind will be remembered at the level of feeling. We all remember emotionally charged events – the time we were attacked by a large dog on our way to school, the day we heard that a school friend had been accidentally killed in a road traffic accident, the excitement tinged with a little fear when we first went on a roller coaster ride. However, to fully understand the relationship between emotion and memory, we need to introduce the hippocampus.

The *hippocampus* is part of the limbic system. It lies close to the amygdala. It appears to be involved in learning and the memory of facts. It is only when the remembered fact is also 'examined' by the neurologically nearby amygdala that its emotional value is recalled. The amygdala has many connections with the hippocampus and other long term memory networks in the cortex. The hippocampus retrieves information and the amygdala determines if that information has any emotional significance. This is why, as we have seen, we have the most vivid memories of things that were emotionally significant at the time in terms of fear or joy, anxiety or desire. Strong emotions are easily evoked by a person or place, even before we have had time to evaluate them in a more conscious, reflective way.

Old experiences therefore emotionally colour new ones. In evolutionary terms, this is adaptive, giving us fast, rough and ready behavioural responses to situations of potential opportunity or danger. But it can also mean that our judgements and reactions can be inappropriate, exaggerated or misleading. A sexually abusive stepfather who wore a certain kind of aftershave is rightly a source of fear for a young girl. But when, as a woman, she smells that same aftershave on an entirely innocent man, her amygdala goes into alarm mode and she feels terror without necessarily knowing why. In this sense, the amygdala is a powerful but generalized, imprecise evaluator of experience that opts for caution.

> When some feature of an event seems similar to an emotionally charged memory from the past, the emotional mind responds by triggering the feelings that went with the remembered event. The emotional mind reacts to the present *as though it were the past*. The trouble is that, especially when the appraisal is fast and automatic, we may not realize that what was once the case is no longer so. (Goleman 1995: 295)

> Such imprecision in, say a squirrel, is fine, since it leads to erring on the side of safety, springing away at the first sign of anything that might signal a looming enemy, or springing toward a hint of

something edible. But in human emotional life that imprecision can have disastrous consequences for our relationships, since it means, figuratively speaking, we can spring at or away from the wrong thing – or person. (Goleman 1995: 23)

The power of very early emotional memories laid down outside language and consciousness is particularly relevant in trying to understand some of the relationship problems experienced by those who suffered pain and hurt, fear and loss in their young childhood. Stimuli in the present go via the senses directly to the amygdala and trigger a powerful experience of the past emotional response. Cozolino (2006: 318) reminds us that the 'amygdala is quick to learn but slow to forget' so that fears are not easily forgotten and will be quickly re-aroused under stress.

For example, a young boy who had suffered physical abuse as a baby remained extremely sensitized to any sudden tactile sensation. In his unconscious mind, any unexpected strong tactile sensation was associated with imminent violence, danger and pain. On one occasion, wearing only lightweight shoes he reacted with panic and terror when unexpectedly he stepped into a deep puddle that was covered with a thin layer of ice. The sudden sensation of cold water on his foot and leg sent the amygdala into alarm mode and he screamed in a state of absolute fear. Under stress, children and adults who have suffered unresolved abuse, neglect and trauma find that the primitive parts of the emotional brain take over from the reflective, cognitive cortex. Under stress – any kind of stress including difficult and tense relationships – these individuals are catapulted into survival mode. They become alert, fearful, tense. Flight, fight and freeze responses predominate as cognition and reflective reason are pushed to the backburner. This can be very puzzling for those on the receiving end of such extreme reactions.

The limbic system and amygdala seem to act as a bridge between the outside world as reported by the senses and the internal world of memory and thought. In this way, an emotional 'value' is attached to the sensation as either positive (approach) or negative (avoid). More generally, the amygdala appears to affect and be affected by what is happening throughout much of the rest of the brain. Neural connections from the amygdala extend in an intricate web to many other parts of the brain. At times of emergency this network of connections allows the amygdala 'to capture and drive much of the rest of the brain – including the rational mind'. (Goleman 1995: 16–17). When we are in the grip of a powerful emotion (sadness, fear, anger), cognition and reflective thought all but cease. All experiences, particularly our dealings with other people, are given emotional value, affective significance and therefore personal meaning.

It is perhaps not surprising then to learn that the amygdala is critical if we are to conduct our social lives competently. It plays a key role in helping us regulate our interpersonal behaviour by triggering feelings of anxiety, attraction, or irritation. Our interpretation of the world around us, suggest Adolphs and Damasio (2001: 43) 'is influenced by mechanisms for assigning emotional and social value, an ability that is clearly essential for survival in a complex social environment . . .'. As a species, we have a highly differentiated set of emotional states that evolved to regulate social behaviour (particularly the social emotions of shame, guilt, jealousy, shyness, embarrassment). Given the particularly complex and critical nature of social life, the highly differentiated character of emotions begins to make sense.

Cortex

Wrapped around and lying on top of the brainstem and the limbic system is the neo-cortex or *cortex* with its familiar wrinkled, deeply folded, tree bark-like appearance. The name cortex in fact derives from the Latin for bark. The cortex makes up 80 per cent of the human brain's volume. Over evolutionary time it grew out of the emotional parts of the brain, thus linking the thinking brain with the feeling brain.

In evolutionary terms the significant development of the cortex is primarily associated with mammals. The cortex is involved in a vast range of functions including thought, perception, language, planning, calculating, purposeful acts, and a constructive and creative approach towards the environment. Interestingly and significantly, many areas of the cortex are taken up with helping us to manage and make sense of our social environment and the part we play in it. If we are to negotiate the subtle and demanding world of other people, we need to build models of some cognitive complexity and sophistication to help us make sense of the interactions between others and ourselves.

In so far as the cortex is heavily involved in helping us manage our social life, it has to be concerned with the emotional side of our nature as most emotions tell us something about our performance in the context of social relationships. In fact, some early speculations suggested that our large brains are primarily the result of us having to process the endlessly difficult and shifting business of relating well and effectively with others. While emotions such as fear, surprise and disgust are basic and easily aroused, emotions that depend on how we evaluate our relationship with others – the higher cognitive emotions – tend to take longer to build up and longer to die away (Evans 2001: 29). These *social emotions* include love, guilt, shame, embarrassment, pride, envy and jealousy. And to the extent that these emotions only arise as we sense how others might be seeing (and evaluating) us, they are the emotions of morality.

In his innovative book, *The Inner Eye* (1986), Humphrey was struck by our interest in what other people might be thinking and feeling. We seem blessed, some say cursed with the skill of social understanding. It was while studying gorillas in Africa that he realized that social life occupies much of the time for most primates, including human beings. He wondered why apes had relatively big brains. After all, on the face of it, their life seemed fairly relaxed and easy. They had plenty of food that required little effort to collect. Gorillas don't move much, preferring to loll around in the company of other gorillas, eating, grooming, mating and rearing their young. Their days seemed pleasant and undemanding. The only thing, thought Humphrey, that seemed to tax them was the behaviour of other gorillas. The only problems for gorillas were, therefore, social. Knowing your place in the dominance hierarchy, who grooms who, where to sleep, can all lead to social challenges or even disputes. Gorillas can also be very co-operative and good social tacticians. So, concluded Humphrey, reading the minds, behaviours and intentions of other gorillas requires a lot of brain power. And what's true for gorillas is probably even more true for humans. The evolutionary advantages of social, co-operative living are huge. Primate brains, mainly composed of the cortex, are big because in part they have to carry out complicated social computations that require enormous neurological computing power. To facilitate social life, we have become natural psychologists.

As a species, we clearly gained an evolutionary advantage as our skills as group living animals increased. Group living led to ever more sophisticated and complex collective behaviour and action, and its associated benefits. And as we relate to many different people, each relationship is also affected and guided by the feelings we have towards each individual. The emotional character of the relationship helps us to negotiate and get right our dealings with one another so that group life and its advantages can operate reasonably smoothly and effectively.

So much of our behaviour with other people is nuanced, and carefully managed and monitored in order to maximize co-operative and reciprocal behaviour. Social skills require us to recognise that other people also have minds with separate thoughts and feelings, and that these govern their behaviour. At the same time, we know that they know we also have a mind full of ideas, interpretations, guesses, beliefs, plans and feelings. Each mind is constantly being affected by and attempting to affect the minds of others, generally to make life work, but also to ensure that one's own interests are likely to be served. Minds, writes Hampton (2004: 51) 'are adapted to other minds'. All of this is a tremendously subtle and demanding business but ultimately it leads to the increased success and survival of our species and our young. Or as Pinker (1997: 193) puts it:

> There's only so much brain power you need to subdue a plant or rock, the argument goes, but the other guy is about as smart as you are and may use that intelligence against your interests. You had better think about what he is thinking about what you're thinking he is thinking. As far as brainpower goes, there's no end to keeping up with the Joneses.

The right side of the cortex, particularly the large pre-frontal cortex (towards the front of the brain above the eyes and therefore known as the orbitofrontal cortex) is closely associated with the processing of emotional experiences. Unlike the amygdala, the pre-frontal cortex handles emotional events in a more considered, reflective, albeit slightly slower fashion. Given time, it might temper the impulsive, precipitate reactions of the amygdala to which it is directly and densely connected, suggesting the importance of the relationship between thought and feeling, cognition and emotion, the cortex and the amygdala.

Emotions give us fast, unconscious reactions as our brains appraise situations outside of our immediate awareness. But one of the evolutionary advantages of the cortex is that it gives us other options based on reflection and analysis. 'One of the reasons that cognition is so useful a part of the mental arsenal', argues LeDoux (1998: 175), 'is that it allows this shift from *reaction to action*. The survival advantages that come from being able to make this shift may have been an important ingredient that shaped the evolutionary elaboration of cognition in mammals and the explosion of cognition in primates, especially humans' (emphasis original).

In practice, the pre-frontal cortex and amygdala generally work in tandem under the more complex conditions of everyday life in which behavioural decisions cannot be made solely by conditioned associations (amygdala) or by exhaustive reasoning (cortex). The cortex's more 'thoughtful' and analytical response is extremely important if the individual is to conduct himself or herself competently or strategically in social situations. Only in emergencies does the more fast acting but less subtle amygdala over-rule the cortex. Under normal emotional conditions, 'the amygdala proposes, the prefrontal lobe disposes' (Goleman 1995: 26).

So, whereas the affective system is busy providing a rapid appraisal and rapid response to stimuli, the 'affective cognitive' system, housed in the pre-frontal cortex, performs a more detailed appraisal of the stimulus, including its relationship to other stimuli and to representations of past experiences. All of this leads to a more modulated, considered response. 'Neural pathways between the amygdala and brain areas involved in cognition allow affect to influence cognition and cognition to influence affect, all of which can occur without conscious awareness' (Taylor and Bagby 2000: 51). Without us realizing it, much of our thinking, particularly in social situations, is constantly being influenced by our feelings. Shimmers of unconscious envy make us more critical than we might realise. Feelings of warmth and sexual attraction lead to praise and support of a colleague. Anxiety causes us to avoid taking on new but challenging tasks, masked even to ourselves by excuses of too much to do and deadlines to be met.

Reason on its own is unlikely to capture the rawness of many situations. Reason alone might leave the individual either in danger or at a social disadvantage. Emotions on their own, except in emergencies, lead to reactions and responses that are too crude. Their lack of refinement and nuance are good for quick, urgent solutions but not much use for more subtle social behaviours. Under everyday and relatively low level arousal, the cortex is able to think about feeling so that the individual's behaviour has emotional intelligence. It is only under emergency conditions that the cortex defers to the limbic system which acts simple and fast. Thought therefore needs to be guided by feeling, but feeling has to be tempered by thought.

Patients who have suffered damage to their right pre-frontal cortex find it difficult to regulate their emotions. The famous case of Phineas Gage illustrates this rather dramatically. Phineas was a well-liked, mild mannered man who worked building railway lines in America during the nineteenth century. One day he was packing dynamite into a drilled piece of rock using an iron rod when the dynamite exploded. The iron bar went straight through the front of his head destroying part of his pre-frontal cortex. Remarkably, Phineas survived the accident but his personality changed. He became aggressive and argumentative. He could not manage his feelings and in the end he lost his job.

Damage to or disease (for example, dementia) of the pre-frontal cortex has a similar affect on most patients. Unsurprisingly, loss of pre-frontal cortical tissue can also impair the ability to recognize the expressions on the faces of other people. This makes interpersonal encounters very difficult. Reading people's emotions from the emotions expressed on their faces is vital to the conduct of social relationships. The pathways between the pre-frontal cortex and the amygdala are particularly active during social interaction. Any loss of emotional sensitivity and intelligence appears to lead to major failures of judgement and relationship competence.

Emotions and the Left and Right Brain

The brain, including the cortex, is divided into two hemispheres – the cerebral hemispheres. Each hemisphere, particularly in the case of the cortex, specializes in different functions. The left hemisphere is more involved with language, logic, cause-and-effect thinking, calculation, analysis and reflection. The right hemisphere is more concerned with non-verbal, emotional processing, facial recognition and interpretation, and more holistic analyses of visual and spacial experiences including art. Linkage between these two hemispheres is most robust in those who have experienced good quality psychological, reflective and emotionally attuned parenting. We have already seen how injury to the right pre-frontal cortex affects the individual's ability to monitor and manage their own and other people's emotions. Indeed, those who have suffered damage here often experience heightened unregulated arousal which they express in strong language and aggressive behaviour. But what if the left hand side of the cortex is damaged?

The left side deals with language and logic, analysis and reasoning. Damage here does not affect the brain's capacity to process emotional experience. However, because it processes speech and language, damage to the left side upsets the individual's ability to talk about feelings even though feelings are consciously experienced. Stroke victims may experience very strong feelings but they struggle to put them into words, adding to their frustration. There is also evidence that the left hemisphere also maintains some kind of inhibitory control over the right hemisphere. Impairments to the functioning of the left hemisphere can lead to a more dominant, emotionally labile right hemisphere in which people appear less emotionally inhibited.

The split into right and left brain functions means that a key task in human development is to integrate emotional and logical processing tasks, that is right and left hemisphere tasks. As we saw in Chapter Four, young children who have experienced emotionally rich environments in which emotions are recognized, understood, named, discussed, talked about, contained and managed, are being helped to integrate their right and left cortex at the neurological level. Secure children who have enjoyed good enough parenting have more complex brains in which dense neuronal connections have been established between the amygdala and the right pre-frontal cortex (or orbitofrontal cortex to be exact), and the right and left sides of the cortex. In this sense, the brain, programmed to make sense of experience, has had good, well modulated and managed emotional experiences of which to make sense. 'Good enough' relationship environments in the early years provide the brain with optimum experiences for robust neurological development.

For infants and young children, the regulation of emotions in close attachment relationships influences the way the brain begins to hard-wire itself to process arousal, feeling and social interaction. 'Human connections create neuronal connections' states Siegel (1999: 85). Attuned communication and good relationships help shape the architecture of our brains.

> During a critical period between ten and eighteen months, the orbitofrontal area of the prefrontal cortex is rapidly forming the connections with the limbic brain that will make it a key on/off switch for distress. The infant who through countless episodes of being soothed is helped along in learning how to calm down, the speculation goes, will have stronger connections in this circuit for controlling distress, and so throughout life will be better at soothing himself when upset. (Goleman 1995: 226)

Neurologically, the dense 'hard-wiring' between the neurons of the limbic system and the orbitofrontal cortex is compromised for children who suffer abusive, neglectful and traumatic early caregiving. When aroused, the developing young brain needs help from comforting caregivers to regulate its distress. Under these managed conditions, the brain learns to make sense of its emotional experiences and in so doing strong neuronal connections develop between the amygdala, the limbic system and the cortex. When help is not available or even worse, when attachment figures are actually the source of the fear and distress, the brain fails to develop strong neuronal links between its emotional and cognitive centres. The trauma experienced in relationship with a hostile carer leads to the release of stress hormones that upset the brain's ability to make connections between the limbic system and the cortex.

It is the strength of the connections between these two parts of the brain – the cortex and the limbic system – that predicts a child's ability to regulate his or her own arousal and distress. This means that when abused, neglected and traumatized children, or adults who have a history of unresolved loss and trauma, experience strong arousal, particularly in the context of stressful relationships, they find it difficult to regulate their emotional distress. In their dysregulated states, they can show uncontrolled anger and aggression, or fear and panic, or despair and hopelessness. With the cortex not in full communication with the amygdala, the monitoring and reflective capacities of the cortex are effectively 'off-line' at times of stress and arousal.

This weakened neurological linkage between thought and feeling, cognition and emotion means that many abused and traumatised individuals have neither the language nor emotional management skills to understand and handle themselves and others well at times of stress and anxiety (Taylor and Bagby 2000: 55). As a result their interpersonal and relationship skills are often poor. They are at risk of mental health problems, including antisocial behaviours and mood disorders. In short, they lack emotional intelligence.

Complex, Integrated Brains

It is now clear that both the cortex and the limbic system, including the amygdala are involved in emotional experience. The more connections between these various parts of the brain, the more individuals are able to draw on both their cognitive, analytical, reflective and emotional resources. Individuals with these highly integrated brains (which are literally more neurologically connected and complex), have more behavioural options to consider in demanding social and relationship-based situations.

This close neurological relationship between the cortex and the limbic system therefore explains why we think and cope more or less well under stress. The prefrontal cortex is the site of short term, working memory. But when we are anxious or emotionally preoccupied (when we feel sad or excited), strong signals from the amygdala interfere with and interrupt normal cognitive activity. Under stress, we talk of 'not being able to keep our mind on the task' and 'not thinking straight'.

The cortex monitors and often puts the breaks on emotional expression and behaviour. It can over-ride, inhibit and repress many of the more primitive responses of the emotional brain. The increasing control of the emotions by the cortex is a distinct developmental feature of human beings. It means that our emotional lives are far more subtle and significant than many other mammals. It isn't that we are less emotional. On the contrary, given our extremely complex social lives, we are probably far more complicated emotional creatures than any other. It is the depth and diversity of our emotional lives that allows us to develop such elaborate and refined social behaviour and interpersonal relationships:

... much of what is special about human cognition and social control of behaviour seems to involve significant inhibitory components above and beyond that displayed by our close genetic relatives. We show greater voluntary control of emotions, particularly sexual behaviour, than any other species; we are able to delay gratification (sometimes for years) in the quest of a goal; we can deceive others or hide our true feelings, often to our political (or simply physical) advantage. Each of these behaviours, while perhaps not unique to humans, reaches its zenith in Homo sapiens and contributes to our success as a species. Each also involves inhibition. Thus, humans apparently increased emotional control relative to other primates is not likely due to a reduction in the role of the limbic system in human behaviour; we remain highly emotional animals. A more likely cause is inhibition from the prefrontal cortex. (Bjorklund and Harnishfeger 1995)

However, at this point a word of caution is necessary. It might be inferred from what has been said that the emotions are primitive and somehow unbecoming to civilized human conduct. In this view, rational thought is seen as superior to emotional experience, that feelings should be distrusted. Although thinking about the emotions in terms of higher and lower brain structure is appropriate, the emotions are not inimical to reason. Although the emotions are clearly different to reason, they actually define our humanity. Indeed, it is difficult to imagine life without the colour and depth and meaning that feelings bring to it. This, of course, is the traditional ground of poets and novelists. The play of emotion in human affairs, how feelings affect behaviour, the highs and lows of simply being, all these continue to be wonderfully explored by the writers of fiction and those who reflect on our shared condition.

To dismiss someone as just being 'emotional' is to forget that it is the emotions that give value or 'valence' to experience. Without feelings, our lives would be flat, monochromatic, and mechanical. We would be socially gauche and incompetent. The limbic system is where emotional experience is generated. As different neurological pathways and circuits are activated under different conditions of arousal, so particular emotional states arise, which when picked up by the cortex are experienced consciously as a feeling.

In many of our day-to-day concerns, feelings outbid thought. Simply trying to think your way out of a strong emotion is very difficult. Feeling sad, frightened, ashamed or jealous can take a powerful hold that is not easily relinquished by considered reflection or careful deliberation. Trying to wish away depression or anxiety is not possible (LeDoux 1998: 19). Each emotion causes us to focus on the thing that preoccupies us and causes the strong feeling. When we are in love all we can think about is the object of our love. Fear makes us focus intensely on whatever is frightening us. This is the way we are made. Emotional intelligence simply requires us to understand the emotional nature of our being.

The Brain's Chemistry

Neurons work by sending electrical signals along their nerve fibres. However, when two nerve cells communicate across the synaptic gap, the brain uses a complex array of chemical messengers known as *neurotransmitters*. Once the chemical message has got across to the next cell, it is converted back into an electrical signal. In effect, the neurotransmitter 'fires' the next cell into either excitement and activity, or just as important, switches it 'off'. But just as things can go wrong with the 'hard-wiring' of nerve cells, so problems can occur with the quality and quantity of these neurochemicals. Neurotransmitter problems and imbalances can lead to a wide range of mental health and behaviour problems including depression and anxiety.

The number of neurochemicals now recognized is considerable but some of the more familiar ones include dopamine, serotonin, acetylcholine, endorphin, and noradrenalin. Serotonin, for example, has been implicated in processes that make us feel positive and bring about a state of well-being. Endorphins, a type of opioid, reduce feelings of pain. They make us feel safe, relaxed and happy. Endorphins are released in both mother and babies when they touch and cuddle, and thus seem to be implicated in caregiving and attachment behaviour. Opioids in general quell the workings of the brain's fear centres including the amygdala.

Endorphins are also released when we are injured. It is one of nature's devices to help us deal with physical insults and traumas. It is hypothesized that those who self-harm experience an endorphin rush which helps them temporarily escape inner shame, fear and despair. Cocaine also suppresses activation of many of those parts of the brain that make us feel wary, anxious, and ashamed. The drug therefore becomes a substitute for the relaxing benefits of enjoying close emotional relationships with others. The attachment is to the drug and not people, particularly at times of anxiety.

Hormones, released by a variety of glands, also act as neurochemicals. They either activate or suppress particular bodily processes. The pituitary gland lies at the centre of the brain and is involved in the control of many other hormonal glands throughout the rest of the body. In its turn, the pituitary gland is largely controlled by the hypothalamus. Adrenaline and cortisol (associated with stress) are two important hormones.

Naturally produced neurotransmitters and hormones affect the way we feel emotionally, psychologically and physically. However, artificial chemicals when introduced into the body can affect the way the brain works and therefore the way we feel. Medicine and pharmacology have taken advantage of this insight to produce a whole range of artificial drugs to treat imbalances in our brain chemistry. Some drugs attempt to increase levels of neurochemicals that are too low in the brain. For example, Parkinson's Disease is partly the result of low levels of dopamine in the brain. Giving patients a drug known as L-DOPA as a pill helps the brain increase its production of dopamine which aids in the improvement of the symptoms of Parkinson's Disease, though not the overall course of the disease. Similarly, low levels of serotonin have been implicated in depression. Drugs that increase the concentration of serotonin in the synapses (for example, Prozac) help reduce feelings of depression; hence they are often described as anti-depressants. More generally, high serotonin levels have been associated with low hostility, low anxiety, improved confidence and an overall sense of wellbeing.

The recreational drug, Ecstasy, targets the neurotransmitter serotonin releasing it in great quantities. Serotonin affects metabolism. Ecstasy can cause hallucinations and a feeling of disembodiment. However, its overriding effect is to make the user feel elated, euphoric and hyperactive. The ability to engage in endless repetitive movements is one of its major appeals to dancers at clubs and raves. Ironically, one of the possible side effects of boosting serotonin output is to damage the nerve endings associated with its production.

Excessive use of ecstasy has been associated with depletion of serotonin and therefore the increased risk of depression.

And yet others drugs act as sedatives. These include alcohol and barbiturates. They induce feelings of sleepiness and reduce alertness and inhibitions. Morphine, including one of its derivatives, heroin, also relaxes people. Feelings of pain diminish. Respiration and breathing slow down. But when taken in excess (overdosing), heroin can cause people to stop breathing altogether leading to inevitable death.

As the name suggests, antipsychotic drugs such as chlorpromazine help reduce some of the symptoms of psychotic illnesses including schizophrenia. One of the effects of antipsychotic drugs is to block the production of dopamine which in excess is thought to bring about some of the symptoms of schizophrenia such as hallucinations.

Thus, as well as prescribed medicines, the other way of affecting brain chemistry is to take non-medicinal drugs – the psychoactive drugs. These include alcohol, nicotine, caffeine, cannabis, amphetamines and heroin. Any one of these drugs will alter our brain chemistry and hence our emotions and mood. That is why, of course, many people take them and why they have been described as recreational drugs. Some drugs act as a stimulant. These include cocaine and amphetamines. For example, amphetamine users can't keep still. Nor can they concentrate. They are easily distracted. 'In many regards', believes Greenfield (1998), 'amphetamine users resemble schizophrenics in that they are constantly at the mercy of the outside world, with no inner resources of mind to assess appropriately what is happening' (p 113).

By helping the brain release more noradrenaline and dopamine, stimulant drugs elevate mood and make people feel more active. When stimulant drugs are taken, the individual feels both excited and physically active. Adrenaline whips people up and thrill seekers crave the highs and buzz that it gives. Dopamine also makes people feel energized and active. Little wonder that people who have low levels of dopamine and adrenaline look to artificial stimulants to give them a 'high'. These are people who are also likely to be risk takers and gamblers. The alternative way to get a thrill, other than use drugs, is to take up an extreme sport. Sky diving or bungee jumping have similar thrilling affects – you get an 'adrenaline rush' – but they avoid the problems associated with drug dependency.

People develop tolerance to many of these non-medicinal drugs so that they need to consume more and more to achieve the same effect. Substance abuse is present when people begin to rely on drugs. Smoking, drinking or heroin begin to play an increasingly critical part in their lives. For many people, it is only a short step from substance abuse to drug addiction. When an individual becomes physically dependent on a drug, they are said to have an addiction to that substance. Not only does the individual begin to show increasing levels of tolerance to the drug, not taking it leads to withdrawal symptoms. These symptoms include cravings, aches, cramp, anxiety, sweating and nausea. Taking the drug removes the affects of withdrawal. The addict once again feels in control, confident and more energetic, ready to face the rest of the day.

Abnormal Brain Functioning and Emotional Dysregulation

When the brain is upset or compromised in its functioning, we experience problems including managing our emotional lives. The upsets disturb the brain's ability to experience, process, monitor and regulate emotions. Emotions that are poorly regulated lead to problem behaviour and mental health problems, relationship difficulties and social stress.

Problems in emotional brain function can be caused by (i) failings at the level of neurons including problems in their layout, density and 'hard-wiring', and (ii) imbalances in the brain's chemistry in which the production of particular neurotransmitters are either too high or too low. These failings and imbalances leading to a variety of mental health and behavioural problems can be diagnosed and explained at a number of levels of dysfunction:

- genetic (for example, genes appear to play a significant part in the risk of developing schizophrenia);
- organic structure of the brain (for example, Attention Deficit Hyperactivity Disorder);
- poor developmental experience (for example, abusive and neglectful caregiving);
- poor environment (for example, high levels of stress);
- injury (for example, damage to the right orbitofrontal cortex leading to a change in personality);

- disease (for example, Alzheimer's disease);
- lifestyle (for example, abusing alcohol and drugs).

Although many of these problems and deficits are irreversible, leaving the individual prey to emotional dysregulation, others can be treated and changed. Many modern medicinal drugs can help the brain produce the missing neurotransmitters such as dopamine in the case of Parkinson's disease or serotonin in the case of depression.

Perhaps surprisingly, changes of environment, particularly the quality of the relationship environment can also bring about changes at the neurological and neurochemical level. Children who have suffered abuse and neglect often fail to develop strong neuronal connections between the limbic system, the orbitofrontal cortex, and the right and left cerebral hemispheres. They therefore have major problems recognizing, understanding and managing their emotions. However, exposure to sensitive, emotionally intelligent care and other therapeutic relationships not only helps these children feel emotionally managed and manageable, it also increases the density of neural connections between the brain's emotional centres. In turn, this leads to improved behaviour and social competence.

Conclusion

The brain is an extraordinarily complex and wonderful organ, but one which is peculiarly sensitive – and therefore potentially responsive – to a wide variety of physical and psychological factors. As we have seen these include hormones, stress, happiness, artificial stimulants and depressants, disease, injury, worry, and relationships. Psychoactive medicinal drugs affecting the brain's neurochemistry have transformed many areas of psychiatry and mental health but perhaps more surprising is recent evidence that sensitive, emotionally attuned, reflective, mind-engaging relationships can also alter brain chemistry and architecture (Cozolino 2006, Siegel 1999). The brain remains 'plastic' throughout life, that is it can re-structure itself in the light of new experience. Relationships present the emotional brain with some of its most powerful experiences. All of this has exciting implications for therapy, counselling and relationship-based social work.

6
Emotions and Physical Health

Introduction

Folk wisdom has always recognized a link between the way we feel and our health, including physical health. We talk about feeling 'sick with worry'. Anxiety gives us a 'knot in the stomach'. It's difficult to relax when we're under stress. For a long time, medicine was perhaps a little sceptical about these old saws, but more recently science has been catching up with the idea that the mind can affect the body. It turns out that the brain and the immune system communicate (Sternberg 2001: xi).

Mind and Body

There are interesting links between how the brain processes and experiences emotion and how this can affect the body. Of course we talk about 'psychosomatic illness', perhaps pejoratively with the implication that weak minds have weak bodies, that for some people who are always complaining that they are unwell, it is merely 'all in the mind'. Psychosomatic illness is based on the idea that conditions of the spirit or mind (*psyche*) can cause diseases of the body (*soma*). However, the modern version explores a far more fascinating connection between mind and body. In particular, the link between mind (made up of thoughts and feelings), brain (made up of neurons, neurotransmitters and hormones), and the body's immune system has created a new health discipline known as 'psychoneuroimmunology' or PNI. In these new sciences, connections are made between neurobiology and immunology, emotions and health, the body and the brain.

For example, feeling anxious does affect how quickly you recover from an illness, injury or operation. Stress does increase the risk of you getting ill. People who generally feel happy and have a positive outlook on life do seem to enjoy better health. And there are good, solid physiological reasons why this might be so. It turns out that the same parts of the brain that control the way we respond to stress are also involved in the way the immune system reacts to disease and infection. Therefore any profession, including social work, which works with people feeling anxious or under stress needs to recognize that emotions affect health and that reducing stress can improve both body and mind.

People react differently to similar experiences. Our personality differences affect the way we each deal with stress and challenge, opportunity and new situations. Both genes and social relationships, particularly between parents and children, influence personality development, and so indirectly also affect our physical health and wellbeing. For example, young children who experience fear, emotional abuse and high levels of stress in relationship with abusive carers might have very depressed immune systems. These psycho-logical differences produce individual emotional reactions which in turn influence mind-body, brain-immune system interaction. Therefore the same external event will be viewed, appraised and emotionally experienced in ways peculiar to each of us individually. This is why some people seem more at risk of poor health than others. Genetic factors, environmental conditions and risky life styles clearly play a major part in our health and wellbeing, but personality factors also seem to interact with each of these components. If we take anxious people, we see that they might suffer high levels of stress if they are in relationship with someone who is easily roused to anger, quick to criticize, and generally unsupportive. Their personal-ity means that they are unlikely to fight back and so they sink into passive despair and experience chronic stress. This cocktail of risk factors is likely to depress their immune system so that they are more likely to suffer infections and illness.

The Immune System

The immune system is a wonderful biological construct that seeks to protect us from disease and infection. The system keeps constant vigilance against invasions from harmful bacteria, viruses and other toxins. The immune system is the result of elaborate interactions between the lymph nodes, bone marrow, spleen, thymus, and other organs. Many of these organs are connected and drained by vessels know as the lymph system that contains a colourless fluid called lymph.

White blood cells, also known as leucocytes, also perform many disease fighting functions. They attack and neutralize harmful bacteria and viruses. There are different types of white blood cells. For example, cells produced by the thymus and secreted into the lymph system are known as T-cells. These cells kill invading organisms that if left to reproduce would quickly make us ill. Antibodies are released into the blood stream by B-cells in the bone marrow. Antibodies attach themselves to foreign bodies in the blood and destroy them. And yet another type of white blood cell known as a phagocyte (from the Greek meaning 'cell eating') surrounds and devours dangerous bacteria and viruses.

In practice, the immune is much more complicated. When the body is under attack, the immune system acts as an elaborate, highly co-ordinated 'defence system' releasing a complex array of cells and antibodies to kill, neutralize and eliminate the disease-creating invaders. However, it is just as important for the body to know how to switch off the immune system once it has done its job. Once it has dealt with the harmful invasion, the body needs an exit strategy. If the immune system isn't switched off, the disease fighting cells and antibodies go on to devour, kill and attack the body's own tissues. This is what happens in diseases where the immune system begins to attack certain cells of the system's own body. This is the case in the autoimmune or inflammatory diseases such as rheumatoid arthritis and multiple sclerosis. When the immune system turns on itself, depending on the nature of the problem, specific tissues might be attacked. So for example, in the case of rheumatoid arthritis the lining tissue of the joints is destroyed. Multiple sclerosis involves the loss of the myelin sheath, a fatty layer surrounding nerve cells, leading to impairment of nerve signalling around the body.

The Stress Response

Individuals experience stress when they feel that the demands being made on them outweigh their ability to cope. It is the subjective *perception* of the demand rather than its objective nature that leads to feeling stressed or not. Two people might react very differently to the challenge of a demanding job or a hostile partner. Lazarus and

Folkman (1984) defined stress as 'a particular relationship between the person and the environment that is appraised by the person as taxing or exceeding his or her resources and endangering his or her wellbeing' (p 18).

Hans Selye is credited with popularizing the word *stress* to describe how our minds and bodies react to pressure when we feel we cannot cope. Stress was, and remains a word used by physicists and engineers to describe what happens when a force is applied to an object. The object will try to resist the force but in doing so, the object will experience stress, distortion and changes in its physical, even chemical structure. Selye (1956) thought the concept of stress lent itself very well in trying to understand biological systems under pressure and tension. He enthusiastically promoted the word until 'stress' was eventually adopted by biologists and psychologists to describe what happens when we feel under physical and personal challenge.

Selye's own experiments with rats led to the idea of stress. He was interested in what might cause rats to develop ulcers. He injected them with various extracts in the hope that he could identify which biochemical substances caused the ulcers. To his initial dismay he found that no matter what substance he injected into the rats, including a neutral saline solution, most of the animals developed ulcers. Eventually he deduced it was the stress of the experiments that was causing the ulcers. The handling by humans, the needles, the injection of a variety of liquids distressed the rats whose bodies reacted in such a way that ulcers were likely to form. Selye than began to notice that most types of stress reduced the health and wellbeing of his laboratory animals including overcrowding, noise, and aggression shown by cagemates. If the stress was prolonged, the rats began to lose weight and became more susceptible to infection, and in some cases they actually died (Sternberg 2001: 64). Rats that suffered chronic stress developed enlarged adrenal and pituitary glands. These glands help in the production of a hormone known as cortisol which floods into the body at times of stress.

This discovery marked the beginnings of many exciting developments in our understanding of how the mind and the body interact. New disciplines emerged including psychoneuroimmunology and health psychology. Social workers pick up the story some way down the line, but if any profession is required to work with people under stress, it is social work. The recipients of their skills and services typically live in poverty or suffer violent relationships; they have to deal with stigma and discrimination; they have to cope with loss and crisis. A basic understanding of how environments affect thoughts and feelings, and how in turn minds affect bodies therefore seems appropriate.

So what are the mechanisms that mean that stress can make you sick? There must be something about how the brain and body react to chronic stress that adversely affects the immune system. If stress impairs the immune system's ability to do its job, we are more likely to get ill, suffer infections and be slow to recover from injury and disease. And as people's psychological strengths and weaknesses vary, based on either their genetic make-up or their nurturing history, their responses to stress will vary with corresponding differences in their susceptibility to ill-health.

When stress is initially experienced – say a partner is threatening to leave, there is a lack of social support, money is in short supply, an eviction notice has been served – the hypothalamus in the brain sends a hormonal signal (CRH) to the nearby pituitary gland. This causes the pituitary gland to produce another hormone (adrenocorticotropic hormone or ACTH) which is released into the blood stream. When this hormone reaches the adrenal glands which wrap round the top of the kidneys (adrenal, from the Latin *ad* meaning towards or near, and *renalis* meaning kidney), they release a third hormone, cortisol into the blood stream. Cortisol acts on many organs throughout the body, including the hypothalamus which when it receives the cortisol signal, shuts down the production of its hormone CTH. 'This ingenious negative-feedback effect of cortisol is what prevents the stress response from spiralling out of control' (Sternberg 2001: 58). This hormonal link between the Hypothalamus, Pituitary gland and Adrenal glands triggered by stress is known as the HPA axis. The adrenal glands also release adrenaline (known as epinephrine in the USA). Adrenaline causes the heart to beat faster, blood pressure to rise, the muscles to tense, blood to flow to the long running muscles, the body to sweat, digestion to stop, libido to disappear, and attention to increase.

In this sense, acute stress triggered by a sudden danger or threat is adaptive. The body rapidly prepares itself for a fight or flight response. And once the threat has gone or the danger avoided, stress levels drop, and the production of cortisol and adrenaline stop.

Remember, it is cortisol that switches off the immune system to prevent it attacking the body's own tissue. So short bursts of cortisol under conditions of sudden stress have little long term effect on the immune system other than to shut it down once it has done its job.

However, *when stress is chronic, the continued production of the stress hormones including cortisol does begin to impair the ability of the immune system to function efficiently*. In effect, the relentless release of cortisol when we feel under long term stress leaves the body with reduced defensive capacity to deal with infection and disease. That is why under severe and prolonged stress we are at increased risk of poor health.

It is entirely adaptive for the stress system to go into sudden overdrive when there is alarm, danger and threat. Fight and flight responses receive the maximum support from the acutely stressed body as it rapidly pumps blood and energy to all the right places. To support the acute need and the stress it induces, all long term, energy demanding systems are temporarily shut down including digestion, growth, repair, sex, and the immune system. The body has a crisis and there is no point investing in processes and functions that are concerned with survival over the longer term.

Unfortunately, human beings have the capacity to worry and this means that the body, to all intents and purposes, can feel under permanent challenge and threat.

> When we sit around and worry about stressful things, we turn on the same physiological responses – but they are potentially a disaster when provoked chronically. A large body of evidence suggests that stress-related disease emerges, predominantly, out of the fact that we so often activate a physiological system that has evolved for responding to acute physical emergencies, but we turn it on for months on end, worrying about mortgages, relationships, and promotions. (Sapolsky 1998: 6)

Thus, stress does not directly make you sick. Stress increases the risk of getting diseases that make you sick. Or, if you have a disease, stress increases the risk of your defences being overwhelmed by the disease. Acute stress is fine if you are in immediate danger or difficulty. Your body rapidly mobilizes for a fight or flight response. However, if you put your heart, blood vessels and kidneys to so much work every time you feel frustrated, angry, or anxious, you increase your chances of heart disease. Those who are prone to worry and suffer chronic stress, and those who constantly feel driven, *hostile* and angry (at work and at home) risk a range of cardiovascular problems including heart attacks (Almada et al 1991). Hostile men are also much more likely to suffer social isolation. This denies them the buffering effects of social support.

> It is very rare . . . that any of the crucial hormones are actually depleted during even the most sustained of stressors. The army does not run out of bullets. Instead, spending so much on bullets causes the rest of the body's economy to collapse. It is not so much that the stress-response runs out; with sufficient activation, *the stress-response itself can become damaging*. This is the critical concept, because it underlies the emergence of much stress related disease. (Sapolsky 1998: 12–13)

Here are some examples of experiments that have tested the relationship between chronic stress, illness and poor recovery.

Cohen et al (1992) hypothesized that the stress emotions would weaken the immune process and increase susceptibility to rhinoviral infections (the common cold). Volunteers were injected with a cold virus. Those who reported high stress in the previous year got infected more readily than those who had experienced low stress. The high stress group had increased susceptibility to the virus because their immune system was weaker. They were also observed to have suffered a loss of T-cell function. This study supports the anecdotal evidence that when we are feeling under stress we are more prone to colds.

In an experiment, Marucha et al (1998) made a tiny cut on the inside of the mouth of 11 dental students. They then examined the speed of healing. Students under stress (about to sit an exam) were compared with students who were experiencing little stress (they were on vacation). On average it took 3 days longer for the wound to heal for the students under stress compared to those on holiday. Extrapolation of these findings suggests that the speed of recovery from illness and injury is likely to be longer when we experience stress.

Although conducted with monkeys and not human beings,

Cohen and colleagues (1991) also found a relationship between social stress and a depressed immune system. Whereas monkeys living in a stable and relaxed social group had healthy immune systems (that is, they enjoyed strong T-cell function), those living in unsettled and socially stressful groups suffered suppressed T-cell function which increased their risk of infection and disease.

Psychology and Immune Functioning:
How Feelings Affect Health and Wellbeing

Our psychological character and personality is a product of our genetic inheritance and social history with parents, family, culture and peers. Different personalities will be more or less prone to stress. There will be people who will feel under stress more readily than others. This will affect not only their mental health but their physical wellbeing. However, some people will be faced with stressful situations that have nothing to do with their personality. Soldiers under enemy fire, a widow whose lifetime partner has just died, a mother whose son is showing signs of attention deficit hyperactivity disorder (ADHD), a family struggling with poverty all experience increased stress. It is still the case that their personalities will affect the way they deal with the stress. We observe how the complex interplay between genes and relationship history creates an individual's psychosocial character which is then faced with the current life stressor. Those with anxious temperaments, or those who as a result of parental rejection suffer low self-esteem and self-efficacy are likely to cope less well with life's hassles and setbacks. Feeling unable to cope, they experience stress which can have a suppressive effect on the immune system thereby increasing susceptibility to illness (Bartlett 1998: 34).

Being a social animal, social change, conflict, breakdown and loss are some of the most stressful experiences that human beings suffer. Simply joining a new social group can be anxiety-provoking. Domestic violence is particularly stressful, not just for the warring partners but also for the children who witness the aggression. Even divorce raises stress levels. Kiecolt-Glaser et al (1987) observed that distressed wives compared to impervious husbands were at greater risk of contracting not just the common cold but also osteoporosis. Our relationship with others lowers stress when it is experienced as loving and supportive, and raises stress when it feels hostile and rejecting. Most of us have experienced stress when we have lost a close relationship through death or rejection. Bereavement makes most of us feel low but those who experience the loss as particularly devastating are most at risk of becoming ill.

The more stressors an individual experiences, the higher the risk of raised stress and depressed immune functioning. Many of social work's service users suffer stress pile-up. Violent partners, low income, behaviourally difficult children, discrimination and social isolation can overwhelm the strongest souls. Social care workers, too, can experience multiple stressors as they try to deal with large caseloads, service users in great need, limited resources, and angry parents. Stress on stress can lead to burn-out when neither the body nor the mind can summon the energy to deal with each day's new challenges. Unrelenting stress can actually change the stress response itself including the body's hormonal systems (Sternberg 2001: 118). Chronic stress can therefore depress libido and the reproductive hormones. It stop women's menstrual cycles, and lowers men's testosterone and sperm counts.

Stress and Coping

Coping refers to behaviour that people use not only to deal well with situations but also to protect themselves from feeling overwhelmed, helpless and stressed by events. The ability to cope acts a protective factor against the stresses and strains of life. When faced with a problem, one or more of the following three protective behaviours might be employed (Pearlin and Schooler (1978):

(i)   modify or change the problematic situations;
(ii)   control the meaning of the experience to neutralize its problematic character; and
(iii) manage the emotional consequences of the experience.

Coping therefore involves cognitive, behavioural, and emotional responses. People who are good at coping and handle stress well tend to use their intellectual, emotional and practical strengths. They analyse problems and break them down into manageable tasks. They plan how to carry out the tasks and in what order. They revise their plans if they hit a brick wall. People who cope are both willing and able to seek social support and help from others.

> We define coping as constantly changing cognitive and behavioral efforts to manage specific external and/or internal demands that are appraised as taxing or exceeding the resources of the person. (Lazarus and Folkman 1984: 141)

Stress, as we have seen, is experienced when the individual feels that they are powerless to deal with the demands of a challenging situation. Individuals vary in terms of at what point they feel helpless and overwhelmed. It is not so much that stress directly causes illness, but by depressing such things as the immune system, it makes us more vulnerable to disease and less able to deal with disease once we are ill.

Psychosomatic medicine is a discipline that considers the effects of stress on individual health. It is as if suppressed and unexpressed emotional troubles manifest themselves as physical symptoms. Being unable to acknowledge or even talk about their feelings, some people's emotions express themselves as physical symptoms. It is the physical symptom that is acknowledged and becomes the nagging concern of the psychosomatic patient, taking many of them with a range of aches and pains, gastrointestinal symptoms, and prolonged fatigue to the surgeries of medical General Practitioners. Both environmental and psychological stress can bring about changes in the body, resulting in illness or physical symptoms. In his comprehensive introduction to 'psychosomatics', Shoenberg (2007) considers a wide range of medical problems that are likely to have a psychosomatic component in their aetiology. He acknowledges that other factors are also likely to be in play in many of these illnesses and symptoms including genes, infection, and immune and environmental problems, but our emotional and mental state can also affect the course of an illness or in some cases actually lead to physical symptoms.

> A psychosomatic illness can be defined as any physical illness in which psychological factors have played a significant role in its precipitation and maintenance and, in certain cases, in its causation as well. In practice, the psychological factors are rarely the

sole or even the dominant ones, except in the case of eating disorders, conversion disorder, hypochondriasis and body dysmorphic disorder. (Shoenberg 2007: 6)

And being psychological in nature, Shoenberg believes that many psychosomatic conditions are responsive to psychotherapy. Mind-body medicine, while not for one moment denying the biogenetic basis of disease and illness, nevertheless sees psychology and psychotherapy playing a useful part in the overall treatment of many conditions ranging from eating disorders to some types of headache, from duodenal ulcers to high blood pressure.

Resilience

Resilience is used as a concept that describes people's ability to deal with stress, pressure and the demands made of them. It suggests the ability positively to adapt to situations of risk that might easily lead to maladjustment in those who are vulnerable (Luthar 2006: 739). Resilience is a complex phenomenon. It is not a unitary concept. No-one possesses across-the-board resilience. Each of us may show varying degrees of resilience in different situations. You may be able to deal well and with skill when confronted by social conflict. However, if your boss pushes too many technical tasks your way, you may quickly feel unable to cope and your stress level begins to rise.

Some resilience factors are genetic. Most of our temperamental traits have a large genetic component. People who by nature are sociable, cheerful, optimistic, plan ahead, and who are good at dealing with new experiences might be expected to show increased resilience in new and complex social situations. Some people are naturally sensitive and easily aroused by stimuli. Physiologically, even small amounts of unexpected stimulation create a big reaction in the form of sudden burst of adrenaline and cortisol. In contrast, other people react to the same stimulus with relatively low increases in adrenaline. In order to get the same level of 'buzz' or thrill, these physiologically under-aroused people need a high levels of stimulation. Kagan (1994) whose work we first met in Chapter Four has been particularly interested in two very basic, but important temperamental types:

Inhibited: This type includes people who by nature are cautious, react to novelty and surprise with restraint, avoidance or distress. Their limbic systems are easily aroused by unfamiliarity. They have a low threshold of arousal. Even small amounts of stimulation produce emotional arousal. They are unlikely to take up bungee jumping or public speaking. In popular parlance they might be described as introverted. If they are exposed to too much novelty and social stimulation they are likely to feel under psychological stress.

Uninhibited. This type includes people who naturally approach new events in a positive, eager fashion without distress. Their limbic systems are not easily aroused. They have a high threshold of arousal. It takes a lot of stimulation to produce emotional excitement. They are more likely to take up extreme sports and be unfazed by performing in public. We often describe these people as extroverts. In their search for stimulation, restless and uninhibited types might place their bodies under high levels of physiological stress.

However, resilience is not just a matter of some naturally given inner strength or the possession of a robust temperament. It is depends on how well people perceive, appraise, approach and tackle stresses and challenges. These qualities are forged in family life and interpersonal experience. Thus, many of life's major resiliences are acquired in the context of close relationships, particularly parent–child and peer relationships.

The protective effects of secure family life and emotional intelligence have been explored by Buckner et al (2003) who found that good emotional self-regulation contributes to resilience as well as sound mental health, particularly in the case of adolescent children raised in poverty. This being the case, Luthar (2006) points out that 'it is far more prudent to promote the development of resilient functioning early in the course of development rather than to implement treatments to repair disorders once they have crystalized' (p 739). Such early interventions include ensuring that children enjoy secure attachments. Emotionally attuned parents promote security. Secure children display high levels of emotional intelligence, and emotional intelligence is a major resilience factor, in part because it predicts social competence and educational success.

Nurture as well as nature therefore plays a key role in resilience formation. Children who have enjoyed secure attachments tend to deal well with stress. In contrast, children who have suffered abuse and neglect experience a surge of stress hormones whenever the environment makes demands of them. Having experienced chronic fear and stress as infants, their stress hormone levels remain high, even under objectively benign conditions. Chronically elevated levels of the hormones associated with stress, including cortisol, increases the risk of poor health.

People who enjoy good social support and close friendships are more resilient. Good self-esteem and self-efficacy (the feeling that with effort you can make a difference, you can bring about change) predict strong resilience. Efficacious people are quick to take advantage of opportunities. They set about trying to solve problems. They seek to bring about changes in their environment to suit their needs and to play to their strengths. In effect, by changing the way things are they create stress-free, conducive environments for themselves (Bandura 1997). Inefficacious people are easily discouraged, fail to tackle the problems, and thereby increase the stressfulness of the situation.

In life, stress of one kind or another is unavoidable. We need to experience stress and arousal to make sure that we are fully engaged with life. We need to monitor problems and recognize opportunities. We also have to note that *the successful resolution of stressful live events has positive effects on confidence, self-esteem, self-efficacy, and sense of personal control*. 'Protection', believes Rutter (1990: 186), 'resides not in evasion of the risk but in successful engagement with it'. If we overcome problems and deal successfully with risk, resilience increases and personal growth is enhanced. For example, Wallerstein (1986) found that 50 per cent of women who had experienced and successfully negotiated marital break up showed long-term psychological improvement. They became more assertive and more realistic. Many improved their self-esteem and embarked on new careers.

Perceived self-efficacy involves judging how capable you are of dealing effectively with a situation. Self-esteem is concerned with judgments of self-worth. There is no necessary relationship between the two. For example, I might judge myself hopeless at ballroom dancing but it does not diminish my self-esteem as I don't invest self-worth in that activity.

The resilience possessed by people who are emotionally intelligent, empathic and have good social cognition seems to come into its own when dealing with people. This means that emotionally intelligent people are likely to cope competently with relationships and so experience relatively low levels of social stress. If in the course of development we feel loved, encouraged to concentrate and persist with difficult tasks, and helped to make sense of our own and other people's emotional and social behaviour, our self-esteem, self-efficacy and social intelligence, and hence resilience are likely to be high.

Feeling in Control

One major component of coping behaviour is feeling in control of the situation. It is loss of control and loss of social support that increase feelings of stress. Being unable to predict a situation or believing that things are getting worse no matter what we do also increase feelings of helplessness. Our psychological character and make-up affects whether or not we feel in control and therefore our susceptibility to stress.

The concept of *locus of control* is viewed by psychologists as an intervening variable. It describes whether an individual feels that events can be controlled by their own efforts or whether control is beyond their personal resources. People who are good at handling many tasks well or dealing with complex challenges seem able to assess situations quickly, break down tasks into manageable chunks, and deal with each task in some order of priority. As a result of their own efforts they feel in control. They are said to possess an *internal locus of control*. The tasks they tackle involve some stress but it doesn't overwhelm them to the point where they feel helpless and adrift. A sense of agency and personal mastery is associated with the ability to perceive situations accurately, analyse challenges strategically and plan responses in the style of a problem solver.

Commitment also acts as a protective factor. People who are curious and become involved with life, whether practically or socially, possess commitment. They see life as meaningful. They accept the world is a changing and dynamic place, never still, and that the best way to live is to embrace this existential flux. Challenges are not threats but incentives. Problems are recast as opportunities. Difficulties are tackled head-on. Life is busy, but stress, low levels of which are vital if you want to stay engaged with the world, is experienced optimally.

It is when we feel helpless and not in control that stress levels continue to increase. A vicious circle sets in. If what happens in a situation is felt to lie outside the control of the individual, they are said to display an *external locus of control*. In the face of a social demand, a practical task, or a decision to be made, they feel passive, impotent, dithering, helpless. They quickly feel under stress and increase the risk of suffering poor health. A sense of powerlessness immobilizes them. They constantly feel that what happens to them is beyond their control. They claim to be at the mercy of forces external to the self and talk about being the victims of bad luck, fate, destiny, or simply say 'that's the way I'm made and there's nothing I can do about. Any effort is futile and a waste of time.' Seligman (1975) describes this approach to life as 'learned helplessness' and it is associated with an increased risk of depression. When people try to cope by avoiding situations, withdrawing from challenges and denying problems, their distress levels actually rise. Life for those who adopt an external locus of control is entirely more stressful.

Loss of control is experienced as particularly stressful. Abused and neglected children, women in violent relationships, adults and children who have suffered extreme fear in war zones all suffer *unpredictable danger*. Worlds in which you have no idea when the next assault or hurt will take place leave you feeling utterly helpless (Howe 2005). Your survival is constantly under threat. Never knowing when the next attack will take place is traumatizing. If you are unable to control these key elements of your environment, you have no choice but to be in 'survival mode' all of the time – watchful, vigilant, anxious, frightened. Stress levels therefore remain permanently high. The physiological responses of those who have suffered trauma, particularly young children, will be altered such that even small amounts of stress will trigger a large hormonal response. Menacing worlds take a heavy toll on both mental and physical health. Often desperate, unconscious measures might need to be taken to try and wrest control, increase predictability and feel safe.

A particularly florid example occurs with what are called *panic attacks*, when the person's anxiety boils out into a paralysing, hyperventilating sense of crisis at some particular moment, often associated with some prior trauma. Another debilitating version of an anxiety disorder is called *obsessive compulsive disorder* (OCD). In this case the person tries to keep the sense of unstructured, menacing panic at bay with an endless variety of reassuring rituals. (Sapolsky 1998: 273, emphasis original)

Feelings of helplessness increase the risk of suffering despair and apathy. In contrast, feeling competent and in control is associated with feelings of well-being. People who try to fathom the nature of their difficulties and don't just give up at the first set back and who don't react fatalistically, these individuals are unlikely to get depressed, unless their explanations and attributions tend towards the negative, in which case they may court anxiety and despair. An internal locus of control encourages active problem-solving. Moreover, people who feel competent and in control actually perceive and experience fewer stressful events. Not only do they have the skills to deal with stress they are also less likely to experience stressful events in the first place.

Stress, Memory and Emotional Arousal

Stress has been found to damage neurons in the brain's hippocampus – a region of the brain involved in laying down memories. People who have suffered severe stress can develop memory problems. The hippocampus's vulnerability to stress can be seen in conditions such as Post Traumatic Stress Disorder in which people have memory problems but suffer no loss of IQ.

In contrast, the amygdala, the fear centre of the brain, which is part of the limbic system, is not affected or compromised by stress. This has an interesting consequence. Events surrounding an experience of fearful, traumatic stress might not be remembered consciously but the amygdala can still be aroused by stimuli that act as reminders of the original trauma. In the presence of the stimuli, the individual will feel great fear and panic, but will be unable to account for it or put the fear into words. For example, a child who has been sexually abused by a cigarette smoking, whisky drinking uncle might become highly distressed whenever she smells tobacco smoke and alcoholic spirits. She feels fear because the amygdala is aroused by the smells but has no conscious memory of the original event because the hyperarousal and trauma damaged the hippocampus's ability to lay down the memory.

As far as is known, stress does not interfere with the working of the amygdala, and . . . stress may even enhance amygdala functions. It is thus completely possible that one might have poor conscious memory of the traumatic experience, but at the same time form powerful implicit, unconscious emotional memories through amygdala-mediated conditioning. And because of other effects of stress . . . these potent unconscious fears can be resistant to extinction. They can, in other words, become unconscious sources of intense anxiety . . . However, there is no way for these powerful implicit memories to then be converted into explicit memories. Again, if a conscious memory wasn't formed, it can't be recovered. (Le Doux 1998: 245–6)

Evolution has built into our biological make-up the emotionally triggered ability to respond to danger without thinking about it first. Anything that hints at past threats causes us to feel fear and adopt a flight, fight or freeze response before we have had time to think about it. According to LeDoux (1998), these unconscious fear memories are indelibly burned into the brain, thus saving us from having 'to learn about the same kinds of danger over and over again' (p 252). Stress can easily re-activate these old fears and anxieties. It is only a problem when these unconscious fear memories begin to affect our day-to-day functioning. This is the case in some forms of traumatic stresses and chronic anxieties.

Happiness, Health and the New Science of Positive Psychology

So minds do affect bodies, and stress can make you sick. The brain, nerve cells, neurochemicals and hormones all become activated by stress and through complex pathways, connections and signalling they change the immune system and the character of its functioning. Change some of the processes and conditions of the brain's complex functioning and you directly affect the immune system. The brain and its processes is the home of our personality and memories, thoughts and feelings. And as our personalities and memories affect what we see, the way we see it, and how we feel, then we can understand how emotional reactions affect the immune system and ultimately our health, for good or ill.

We have seen that many of our most powerful emotions, both positive and negative, are experienced in our relationships with others. Negative emotions are stressful and can undermine our health. Good social relationships and strong social support create positive feelings, lower stress and promote health and wellbeing. People who enjoy warm friendships and can turn to others at times of need are said to be socially 'embedded'. They are 'connected' to others and the soothing social supports they offer. Cohen et al (1997) have even shown that individuals who enjoy rich and varied social networks are less likely to get ill.

Happy people report fewer aches and pains than those who say they are in a sad mood. Optimists and those who are happy have more robust immune systems. They enjoy better health. They have more social supports. And of course, they are more likely to adopt life styles that are healthy, augmenting their already sound immune functioning. Happy people are less likely to smoke, or abuse alcohol and drugs. They tend to be more physically active, and activity itself promotes the release of brain chemicals that further increase our feelings of happiness. One of the evidence-based recommendations for treating depression is take more exercise.

This interest in happiness and wellbeing is part of the new science of positive psychology. Traditionally, so much of psychology was concerned with minds not working well. In reaction, Seligman (2003) was one of the first to explore the psychology of happiness, how we flourish, how we experience 'the pleasant life'. Positive psychologists aim to understand what makes us happy, and how happiness affects health, both physical and mental (Argyle 2001; Csikszentmihalyi 1998).

The classic 'Nun's Study' nicely captures the health benefits of enjoying a positive outlook on life. Nuns who entered convent life in the 1920s with a very positive, joyous emotional outlook were compared with those who joined in a somewhat more serious, emotionally flat state of mind. When examined over their lifetimes, the emotionally positive nuns lived on average nine years longer than their more negative sisters (Danner and Snowdon 2001). Happy people and those who laugh do indeed appear to have a higher chance of living longer. 'Being happy', says Martin (2005: 31), 'is seriously good for your health'.

It is interesting to note how infectious laughter can be. Whether or not we know what other people are laughing at, we tend to smile and even begin to laugh ourselves. Whether it's other people cheering, giggling or laughing we very quickly find ourselves joining in. Our brains are programmed to mirror other people's behaviours and actions which we then mimic. 'Mirror neurons' are activated when we watch someone else behaving or expressing an emotion (Rizzolatti et al 1999). Mirror neurons are also involved whenever we attune to the emotional condition of another. As we unconsciously mimic, both at the neurological and behavioural level, the behaviours and feelings of other people, we understand their experience from our own mental insides. We have an *as if* feeling whenever unconsciously we mimic the action, facial expression, intention, or movement of the other (Damasio 1999). Mirror neurons lie next to motor neurons so that firing in one has the potential to excite the other. We wince when we see someone accidently hit their thumb with a hammer, or we subtly mimic the actions of a man who is struggling to lift a heavy weight. These are known as *resonance behaviours*.

Neurological and behavioural mirroring seem to be particularly pronounced in the case of laughter, and with people we like or fancy. Being in the company of happy people is both infectious and good for our health. Similarly, when people flirt with each other, they begin, unconsciously, to copy the other's behaviour and speech patterns. Laughter and most of the positive emotions promote social bonds and increases our sense of belonging. When we laugh, endorphins, opiate-based neurotransmitters, are released in the brain. Endorphins make us feel good; they give us a 'high'. They inhibit activation of the amygdala and so reduce feelings of anxiety. When we have had a good laugh, we feel better, more co-operative, accepting, genial and generous (Provine 2000). In a very real sense, both psychologically and physically, laughter can be the best medicine.

Conclusion

Running throughout this chapter is the insight that many aspects of our health and wellbeing require us to feel involved, recognized and connected with other people, particularly at the emotional level. People who enjoy strong social relations also tend to possess good emotional intelligence. The risk for those whose emotional intelligence is underdeveloped is an increase in social isolation. Those who feel lonely experience more stress and poor health. Some of the benefits of group support and therapeutic group work lie in the raised positive emotions that can be experienced when we feel connected and understood by others. Spiegal et al (1989) found that positive therapeutic group support in which seriously ill patients could express their feelings had distinct health benefits. Although group support is unlikely to cure the actual illness, it can help patients live and cope better with their condition.

Emotions, their expression and the social signals transmitted by our senses allow us to communicate our feelings to other people. This facilitates social and group action. Anger, fear and disgust warn of danger. Smiling signals safety, affection, acceptance. So although physically we end where our bodies end, by expressing feeling we literally affect and connect with the bodies and minds of other individuals (Sternberg 2001: 141). Our warmth and emotional availability lend friends confidence and energy. With our help and co-operation, situations feel less stressful. But if we are rejected and greeted with hostility, our sense of isolation and danger increase. Attack by others or feeling outside the group increases stress and anxiety.

We are all subtly connected to other people via our senses, our emotions and our minds. Because we are a social species embedded in a matrix of relationships, to an extent our psychological and physiological selves are socially constructed. Health and illness therefore have a distinct psychosocial dimension. The negative strains and emotional supports that we experience in day-to-day social interactions play their part in sickness and in health. We constantly strive to keep a balance between our need to feel competent and in control, autonomous, and socially embedded. Mental health and physical wellbeing lie in getting this balance right.

7
Emotions and Mental Health

Introduction

Emotions play a central role in the way we psychologically experience ourselves and the manner in which we conduct social relationships. They help organize our thoughts and actions. They guide our behaviour and allow us to meet the challenges of everyday life. The ability to understand and regulate our own and other people's emotional states and the ability to manage relationships well defines much of what it is to be mentally healthy. Individuals with integrated brains in which the complex relationship between thought, feeling and behaviour is recognized and handled well are generally good at managing social interaction. Emotionally intelligent people tend to enjoy good mental health. Those who cannot regulate their emotions become slaves to them (Salovey and Mayer 1990: 201). They mismanage relationships and are more likely to suffer poor mental health.

Emotions Awry

If we are a socially based species, one that negotiates relationships using emotions as interpersonal radar then, suggest Kring and Werner (2004), it isn't surprising that 'emotion disturbances figure prominently in many different forms of psychopathology. By one analysis, as many as 85% of psychological disorders include disturbances in emotional processing of some kind' (p 360). If we think about many mental health disorders, they are partly defined by emotions being in excess (for example, too much anger, anxiety or fear) or in deficit (too little joy) or muddled and incoherent.

The idea that 'madness' lies in emotions being wildly out-of-control has been around for a long time. When we are no longer susceptible to the regulatory influences of others, our behaviour is less predictable and society gets anxious. Those who are sad and withdrawn, angry and violent, frightened and in torment are soon identified as souls in trouble. Something should be done for them or done about them.

> [O]ur emotions can get us into trouble. When fear becomes anxiety, desire gives way to greed, or annoyance turns to anger, anger to hatred, friendship to envy, love to obsession, or pleasure to addiction, our emotions start to work against us . . . mental problems to a large extent, reflect a breakdown of emotional order. (LeDoux 1998: 20)

If we are to conduct ourselves with social skill and competence, then we need to regulate our emotions and their expression. This involves knowing what emotional mood we are in, what has caused it, how it is affecting us, how we are expressing our feelings, and how other people might be perceiving and reacting to that expression. The emotionally intelligent individual is both aware of and monitors the cause, intensity and display of feeling. The more self-aware the person, the greater their ability to modify both the internal experience of the emotion and its external display. So, for example, we don't make jokes if someone is feeling very cross and dissatisfied with our decision. These self-controlling skills are only gradually learned by children. Giggling when a pompous uncle visits may not be appreciated by parents anxious to make a good social impression.

A preliminary analysis of some of the more common psychological disturbances and mental disorders immediately shows that the presence of emotion-related symptoms forms a key part of psychiatric recognition and diagnosis. Emotional dysregulation underpins much of psychopathology. It is difficult to reason with people who find themselves in the grip of powerful feelings and unregulated emotions. The smooth conduct of social relationships is not easily achieved by those who are depressed or anxious, angry or intemperately euphoric.

Taking an emotional perspective, a condition is typically defined by a particular emotion being present in excess, while other more socially expected emotions are absent. So, depression is characterized by overwhelming feelings of despair, hopelessness and sadness. Depression is one of the most widespread and common mental health concerns. A diagnosis of bipolar disorder is applied when an individual alternates between depressed and manic episodes in which emotions run high and the patient is wildly optimistic, expansive, impatient and sometimes irritable. Anxiety disorders cause people to feel excessively agitated and distressed. For example, agoraphobics feel intense anxiety in busy and unbounded social situations. A range of mental health and behavioural problems cluster around anger and aggression including conduct disorders and antisocial behaviours. Borderline personality disorder is present in those who cannot control their emotions, switching unpredictably between intense displays of aggression, need, shame, impulsivity, despair, boredom, and a wish to self-harm.

We now expand this understanding of mental health problems in which emotions might be dulled, out of balance, or out of control. Health and social care professionals will be working routinely with people many of whom will be affected by one or more of these states. Linking these diverse categories is the underlying theme of the emotions being out of kilter. Understanding this element of people's mental health should give practitioners an insight into how delicately we are all poised between equanimity and anguish. Recognizing this shared fate encourages emotionally intelligent professionals to practise with compassion.

Schizophrenia

Although the major psychoses, such as schizophrenia, are not generally considered simply as problems of emotional regulation, nevertheless the illnesses do upset people's emotional experience. Schizophrenia is an illness in which perceptions and thought processes become disturbed and disordered. Both genetic and environmental risk factors are implicated in the development of schizophrenia resulting in pathological neural development and problems with brain chemistry. Schizophrenia is in fact a broad syndrome in which different types of schizophrenia are identified. For example, paranoid schizophrenia is diagnosed in cases where individuals hear voices, feel persecuted, or might have delusions of grandeur in which they believe they are Jesus or God. 'I thought the voices I heard were being transmitted through the television', said James. 'The voices kept telling me to do things like warn everybody that the government was about to release a poisonous gas through the water pipes.

I thought my house was being bugged by the government so I had to be extremely careful what I said. My thoughts kept racing and racing.' In contrast, people who suffer catatonic schizophrenia might remain motionless, adopting odd postures, for long periods of time, saying nothing.

In general, there is evidence that schizophrenia patients tend to be less emotionally expressive than those who do not have the illness. The voice becomes flat. The face loses mobility. Emotions are experienced but not communicated. Kring and Werner (2004) also report that schizophrenia patients are less likely to differentiate between emotional states. This impairs their ability to regulate arousal and conduct themselves appropriately in social relationships.

There is also evidence that the families of some patients with schizophrenia are characterized by high levels of stress, tension, conflict, poor communication, disapproval, high rates of criticism, intrusion and over-involvement in each other's private business (all described as high *expressed emotion* or EE). Individuals trying to recover from schizophrenia are four times more likely to relapse when they return to families with high 'expressed emotion' compared to those who return to those with low 'expressed emotion' where recovery rates are much better (Brown et al 1962). There is, of course, also the possibility that individuals with schizophrenia are very difficult to live with; that is they generate stress, conflict and tension in their families.

Alexithymia

A problem for individuals and society is when people seem not to experience, express or articulate emotions with any great facility. As emotional literacy and social competence go hand in hand, to feel emotionally empty or confused will lead to relationship difficulties. Somatization and alexithymia are two conditions loosely connected around the theme of dulled emotional awareness.

Alexithymia is a condition in which the individual has difficulty recognizing and finding words for their feelings. As a result they have problems talking about their emotions. They occupy the low end of the emotional intelligence spectrum.

The word alexithymia is derived from the Greek: *a* meaning a 'lack', *lexis* meaning 'word', and *thymos* for 'emotion', hence literally a lack of words for feelings. People who suffer the condition typically lack imagination. Unable to express or articulate feeling, they use direct physical action or bodily behaviours for emotional expression. Not surprisingly they respond poorly to insight-oriented psychotherapies. Lacking emotional awareness, they report an absence of inner experiences (Taylor and Bagby 2000: 41–2). They rarely remember dreams, and their thinking is concrete and lacks emotional colour. Their behaviour is guided by rules, regulations and the expectations of others rather than by their own feelings, wishes, and personal values.

According to Parker (2005), the clinical implications of these inabilities are vast, 'since they have been associated with a variety of clinical disorders, and anxiety disorders; within various non-clinical populations, these abilities have been linked with a variety of health, lifestyle, and interpersonal problems' (p: 272). Many alexithymic individuals develop psychosomatic symptoms and often engage in binge eating, alcohol abuse and other compulsive behaviours seemingly in an attempt to regulate distressing inner states. Unable to access an inner life of feelings, these patients are preoccupied with physical symptoms. They relate to others without displays of affect. Theirs is a literal world.

Alexithymia can sometimes be associated with Post Traumatic Stress Disorder. There is certainly a tendency to give external expression to inner states through *somatisation*, that is the symptoms are manifested in the body and its functions (for example, stomach pains, bowel problems). If emotional feelings cannot clearly be recognized but there is a sense of unease, there is a tendency to 'over-read' physical sensations, exaggerating them out of proportion to their actual significance leading to hypochondria and eventually real symptoms in the form of 'somatization' – the bodily expression of psychological states.

> It is not surprising that alexithymia has been conceptualized as one of several possible personality risk factors for a variety of medical and psychiatric disorders involving problems in affect regulation. For example, hypochondriasis and somatization disorder might be viewed as resulting, at least in part, from the alexithymic individual's limited subjective awareness and cognitive processing of emotions, which leads both to a focusing on,

and amplification and misinterpretation of, the somatic sensations that accompany emotional arousal. (Taylor et al 1997: 31)

In terms of visits to the doctor, alexithymics make greater use of the health services as they tend to somatize their distress. Misunderstanding the nature of the problem can lead to inappropriate medical treatments. Treating alexithymia is difficult. There is a need to help the patient 'to elevate emotions from a level of perceptually bound experience (a world of sensations and action) to a conceptual level (a world of feelings and thoughts) where they can be used as signals of information, thought about, and sometimes communicated to others' (Taylor et al 1997: 252). They need to recognize and correctly label emotions, learn to differentiate among different emotional experiences, and learn better to communicate these feelings to others. However, most people with alexithymia find any discussion about emotion boring, even frustrating. They find close emotional relationships (for example, with the therapist) difficult; even anxiety-provoking. It is a long, slow process trying to help people with the condition connect with their own and other people's feelings.

Autism and Autistic Spectrum Disorders

Children and adults on the 'autistic spectrum' have impaired social functioning and interpersonal communication. They display obsessional behaviours. They like sameness and routine. For example, a child might spin the wheels of a toy car repeatedly for hours on end. Many have learning difficulties and never manage speech. And yet others develop extraordinary skills in a very defined area such as mathematical computation, drawing or knowing all there is to know about a very specific, esoteric subject such as a railway timetable. It is now generally accepted that autism is a neurodevelopmental disorder with characteristic cognitive deficits and a *strong* genetic influence. (Baron-Cohen 1995; Frith 1991; Happé 1996; Rutter 2006)

As we saw in Chapter Four, one of the defining features of autism is the limited ability of children and adults to be aware that other people have minds and mental states and that what goes on in other people's minds is useful knowledge if you are to conduct yourself competently in social relationships. Baron-Cohen (1995) called this deficit 'mind-blindness'. This would include difficulty in recognizing, or indeed being interested in other people's emotional states. This being the case, Baron-Cohen (2004) also refers to autism as an 'empathy disorder'. Autistic children typically make little eye contact, and show little of the facial and emotional expressions and gestures that normally help regulate social interaction – looking apologetic if you have done something wrong, trying to cheer someone up if they are looking sad. People's thoughts and feelings are complex, unpredictable and ultimately unknowable and perhaps best avoided. Computers, timetables, and mathematics are logical, systematic, predictable, and knowable. They afford feelings of familiarity, control and safety, and therefore might be a source of comfort for those at the higher functioning end of the autistic spectrum (Baron-Cohen 2004).

Little wonder then that the buzzing, confusing world of people and relationships is so puzzling and distressing. This lack of emotional empathy does not mean than those with autism don't experience emotions. Certainly frustration, anger and distress is felt if a routine is upset, or familiar order breaks down. This might explain why people with autism and autistic spectrum disorder try to regulate their emotions by trying to control their environment, which might include people and what they do. It is not surprising that many adults who have suffered a lifetime of not quite fitting in, being perceived as odd, possibly experiencing bullying and rejection, suffer depression. They recognize that they don't fit in, or that socially they get things wrong, but they don't quite understand why, or what it is that other people are doing that allows them to be so effortlessly fluent when conducting social relationships. Knowing how to behave in social situations is a huge burden. What comes naturally to most children and adults is a constant struggle for individuals with autism, including those with Asperger Syndrome.

Loss, Grief and Mourning

Our interdependence with others means that we are psychologically vulnerable to the loss of any close relationship. We are defined by our relationship with others. Feelings of safety, acceptance, worth, connectedness and love are experienced as we interact with partners, family and friends. Loss of any one of these social bonds fractures our sense of self. We might feel exposed and vulnerable without our life-long partner. To whom can we now turn to at times of need? Without the love and admiration of others, our self-image and worth is diminished. Bowlby (1969, 1979, 1980) recognized the importance of loss and separation in understanding the origins of people's grief and pain, anger and depression. Loss can be caused by death, aban-donment, withdrawal and rejection. Loss triggers sadness. Loss is stressful.

Bereavement can affect both physical and mental health. Those who have recently lost a close partner are at increased risk of depres-sion and physical illness. However, these upsets can be mediated by other factors, particularly the social support of others.

Loss and grief as psychological phenomena were first looked at scientifically by Lindemann (1944). He studied people's reaction to loss after a disaster. In Boston, Massachusetts, two Catholic colleges were well known for their football rivalry. In the autumn of 1942, Holy Cross beat Boston College. After the game many people went to the local Coconut Grove Nightclub to celebrate. In the middle of the party, a busboy lit a match while trying to replace a light bulb. He accidently set a decorative palm tree on fire. Almost immediately, the whole nightclub was engulfed in flames. Nearly 500 people died. Lindemann, a psychiatrist, and his team worked with the grieving relatives. In 1944 he wrote a classic paper based on his work with 101 of the bereaved patients. He identified a number of features typical of normal grief:

- somatic or bodily distress of some type;
- preoccupation with the image of the deceased;
- guilt relating to the deceased including circumstances of the death;
- hostile reactions;
- the inability to function as one had before the loss.

Our thoughts, feelings, behaviour and bodies are all affected by grief. Matters can get complicated when our relationship with the lost other was difficult, ambiguous or unresolved in some way. Some people experience anger, others guilt. In the case of a violent or undermining relationship, there might even be a feeling of relief and emancipation. There might be hurt and anxiety trying to imagine how life can possibly be lived without the dead husband, rejecting lover, deceased child. There will be loneliness.

Over the years a general grief and mourning cycle has been worked out. Not everyone goes through all stages; not everyone goes through them in the same order. The basic stages include: protest (loss), followed by yearning and despair (mourning), leading to detachment (a form of defensive protection). The broad features of this cycle seem universal:

- shock and disbelief, even denial;
- confusion of thought and difficulty concentrating;
- numbness;
- anger and protest;
- yearning and pining;
- depression;
- disorganization of thought, feeling and behaviour;
- preoccupation thinking about the lost other, including how to recover them;
- physical reactions;
- social withdrawal;
- adjustment, re-organization, restitution and a gradual return to normal functioning: acceptance, resolution and re-integration.

In the early stages of grief, many people experience strong somatic reactions. They might feel knotted and hollow inside. The psychological pain can be palpable. People 'ache' with longing. The throat feels tight. Tears come suddenly and desperately. There is over-sensitivity to loud noises and bright lights. Some people suffer 'depersonalization', a feeling that everything seems unreal and distant, including the self. Appetites are lost and sleep is disturbed. Apathy and slowness of movement can also characterize the behaviour of some bereaved people, while others feel restless.

The length of the overall grief and mourning cycle can vary enormously from weeks, months to years. A few people get stuck and can't move on. Mourning rites and the gathering of friends and family can help people through the early stages. The way people mourn tends to be a product of their relationship history and the quality of their current relationships. Unresolved grief is more likely to occur when the relationship between the bereaved and the deceased was very close, dependent, conflicted, or ambivalent; or when the death was sudden; or if the bereaved has a history of depression. Grief can feel particularly intense if the loss is compounded by other losses and setbacks. Karl lost a job he liked then fell into debt. The stress this caused put a strain on the relationship with his long-time girlfriend. Not long after they separated under less than happy circumstances, Karl's mother died. After a highly distraught initial reaction, Karl fell into a prolonged state of depression.

Looked at from an attachment perspective, the grief and mourning cycle is based on the double blow that children and adults experience when the attachment figure, the supportive partner, or the close friend in whom one confides is lost. Feeling distressed and insecure normally activates attachment behaviour which entails seeking out the loved one for protection, comfort and understanding. But of course, this person, whose loss has caused the distress, is no longer available to help resolve it. This combination is particularly upsetting and can have its most traumatic affects on young children, particularly if the quality of care by those remaining is poor. Fraiberg describes the child's personality as *interpersonality*. 'Therefore, when that bond is broken, the very structure of the personality is endangered' (cited in Fahlberg 1991: 143).

There are wide cultural differences in the way that grief is experienced and dealt with. One extreme is represented by societies in which there is the feeling that grief should be contained, at least in public, and the bereaved should try and move on with their lives as soon as possible and leave their dead behind. At the other end of the cultural spectrum are societies that accept that the dead are always with us, that the bonds that tied us to loved ones don't simply go away. Here, grief is encouraged and its expression respected. Loss needs to be acknowledged and talked about. This approach sponsors customs that allow for the memory of the deceased relative or friend to be incorporated into the rhythms of life. The anniversary of the death is an occasion for fond remembrance and re-engagement. To the extent we experience ourselves in a matrix of close relationships, these practices allow the self to preserve a degree of coherence and continuity.

Major Depression

The main diagnostic features of depression are familiar to most of us: prolonged sadness and depressed mood, anxiety, guilt, and perhaps irritability. Feelings of hopelessness and worthlessness are common. People with depression often disengage from social life. There is a loss of interest in everything and everybody. Apathy is high. Concentration is low. Libido disappears. Sleep rhythms are upset and although people often wake early, they feel tired and without energy. They tend to perceive and attend to the more negative aspects of thought, memory and events. This creates a negative cognitive bias and negative thinking. Once in this loop of negative emotions, it is difficult to take control and regulate them. Trapped in a round of negative thought, sufferers develop a negative view of self, the world and the future (Beck et al 1979). Some sufferers will think that suicide is a better option than living a life that seems pointless.

Depression is one of the most common psychopathologies. In any normal population, prevalence rates run at around 6 per cent. Twice as many women as men are diagnosed with depression. Stress certainly seems to play a part in the onset of the illness. Given that women experience more stress in their lives than men (they suffer reduced status, power, income, and locus of control), their higher rates of depression might not be so surprising.

Major depression is not simply feeling sad. It is a serious mental illness. The following quote from the eminent biologist Lewis Wolpert gives a sense what it feels like to be in the trough of a deep, major depression:

> It was the worst experience of my life. More terrible even than watching my wife die of cancer. I am ashamed to admit that my depression felt worse than her death but it is true. I was in a state that bears no resemblance to anything I had experienced before. It was not just feeling very low, depressed in the commonly used sense of the word. I was seriously ill. I was totally self-involved, negative and thought about suicide most of the time. I could not think properly, let alone work, and wanted to remain curled up in bed all day. I could not ride my bicycle or go out on my own. I had panic attacks if left alone. And there were numerous physical symptoms – my whole skin would seem on fire and I developed

uncontrollable twitches. Every new physical sign caused extreme anxiety. I was terrified, for example, that I would be unable to urinate. Sleep was impossible without sleeping pills: these only worked for a few hours, and when I woke up I felt worse. The future was hopeless. I was convinced that I would never work again or recover. There was a strong fear that I might go mad. (Wolpert 1999: vii)

Modern explanations of the causes of depression implicate genes, poor relationship histories, and current life stressors. Some people seem more genetically vulnerable to depression. As we saw in Chapter Five, the neurotransmitter serotonin is thought to help regulate other neurotransmitter systems in the brain. Low serotonin activity disrupts the activity of the other neurotransmitters and can lead to depression. Modern medicine's understanding of the role of neurotransmitters in depression has allowed the development of a range of anti-depressive drugs many of which help the brain increase serotonin levels. Particular genes are involved in the production or not of serotonin. According to the work of Caspi et al (2003), people who inherit two of the short forms of a particular gene (known as 'serotonin transporter gene 5-HTT') are at increased risk of depression *but only if they meet significant life stressors*. Depression therefore requires a complex interaction of genes and environment, nature and nurture before it becomes manifest. To an extent, supportive environments (a caring partner, adequate income, good friends) and low stress can protect those who are genetically at risk from becoming depressed.

The original work of Brown and Harris (1978) in Camberwell in East London examined the psychosocial factors that appeared to be playing a part in the onset of depression. They considered the effects of severe life events on depression as well as the stress-buffering effects associated with current life circumstances, particularly the protective value of a warm, confiding relationship. In their study population of working class women they found a greater prevalence of depression amongst those who had the following vulnerability factors:

- loss of mother before the age of 11 by death or long term separation;
- the absence of a reliable, warm and protective caregiver after the loss of the mother;

- lack of paid employment outside the home;
- three or more children under 14 years of age still living at home;
- current lack of an intimate, confiding relationship.

Brown (1998) has continued to refine his psychosocial model of depression. With colleagues, he has added to the above list of vulnerability factors: feeling trapped in a loveless marriage with a needy, feckless and unsupportive partner; and in the case of women who enjoyed happy marriages, the loss of a husband through death. Feelings of 'entrapment' and 'humiliation' cause despair. Partners who leave you for another, who belittle you, who continue to make impossible demands undermine the core sense of self. Low self-esteem saps personal worth and belief. When people feel powerlessness, defeated, and lack the means of escape from unloving, demanding relationships, depression is likely. The feeling that you are unable to control your world at the deepest levels of safety, self-worth, joy, and hope is frightening and profoundly depressing. It calls into question the very purpose of one's life.

It seems that the interaction of a variety of psychosocial factors including (i) early loss, poor care and emotional deprivation in childhood, and (ii) later life stressors, particularly feelings of entrapment and lack of control, increase the risk of depression. More specifically, adults who suffer violence and rejection in childhood without the benefits of an alternative protective relationship are at particular risk.

Brown (1998) summarized his position arguing that genetic and biological risk factors are important, but they are best seen as contributing to variability in risk within populations which is largely driven by psychosocial factors. His study of life events has been critical in developing this radical social perspective. He concludes:

> . . . that it is not improbable that most cases of depressive disorder result from a failure to meet goals derived from evolutionary-based needs such as being admired, forming friendships, having a core adult attachment figure, having children, and so on. These goals are almost entirely social in nature. (Brown 1998: 369)

Cognitively, stressed and depressed people hold distorted beliefs that there is no control or outlet for their despair. They show 'learned helplessness'. On the affective level, there is anhedonia – the inability to feel pleasure. Behaviourally there is psychomotor retardation – sufferers move slowly and with seeming effort. 'On the neurochemical level, there are likely disruptions of serotonin, norepinephrine, and dopamine signalling; physiologically, there are alterations in, among other things, appetite, sleep patterns, and sensitivity to the glucocorticoid system to feedback regulation' (Sapolsky 1998: 258). It is the combined presence of these cognitive, emotional and behavioural deficits, coupled with the underlying imbalances in brain chemistry that we call depression.

Bipolar Disorder

Men and women are equally at risk of developing bipolar disorder. The illness describes periods of depression punctuated by episodes of mania in which the individual experiences intense euphoria, optimism, delusional grand designs, and irritability. The condition used to be known as manic depression.

Although modern diagnostic manuals require at least one burst of mania to be present, depression is not absolutely necessary although many bipolar disordered patients do experience depressive symptoms. The disorder describes those who cannot regulate intense experiences of either positive or negative arousal. This creates swings in mood cycles that can interfere with daily functioning and put a strain on relationships. Feelings quickly get out of hand. Suicide rates amongst those with bipolar depression run at 10 to 20 times the rate found in the normal population, although this still only represents 0.4 per cent of all those with the diagnosis.

There is still uncertainty about the exact cause of the illness but high levels of adrenaline and serotonin are reported during manic episodes which then drop to low levels during depressive phases. Abnormalities in brain organization have also been suggested. There is evidence that genes and heritability play a part. Well over half of people diagnosed with bipolar disorder have a relative who has suffered either major depression or bipolar disorder suggesting a strong genetic predisposition particularly if environmental stressors are also experienced.

It has been observed that there is some association between bipolar disorder and creativity. It has been observed that Virginia Woolf, Ernest Hemingway, Sylvia Plath, William Blake, Tchaikovsky,

Vincent van Gogh and John Ruskin amongst many others were probable sufferers of the illness. There seems to be something about the way those with manic depression experience the world that gives them a deep insight into the highs and lows of our emotional being. They seem able to pierce the fabric of life when their gaze is intense and their levels of energy are on full power. There is evidence that emotional sensitivity, risk taking and willingness to experiment are greater. Everyday conventions which limit experience and reach are ignored leaving the individual gloriously free to explore without inhibition the world unbounded.

However, the disorder should not be romanticized. When individuals are suffering the extremes of their illness – depression or full-blown mania – they are unlikely to be productive let alone creative. Some people in their manic episodes adopt an extravagant, reckless lifestyle, spending money they don't have on clothes or cars. Many are disruptive, talking excessively day and night, executing increasingly out-of-control plans. They teem with ideas, most of them crazy. Thoughts race in the mind. Judgements are poor and behaviour can be indiscreet. Sleep is reduced, and attention spans are short. Some people become aggressive if their wild plans are thwarted. Episodes of mania can last a few days or up to several months. But when the manic episode is lost, many individuals collapse into a profoundly depressed state. Jamison, a psychiatrist, describes the manic phases of her bipolar disorder:

> There is a particular kind of pain, elation, loneliness, and terror involved in this kind of madness. When you're high it's tremendous. The ideas and feelings are fast and frequent like shooting stars, and you follow them until you find better and brighter ones. Shyness goes, the right words and gestures are suddenly there, the power to captivate others a felt certainty. There are interests found in uninteresting people. Sensuality is pervasive and the desire to seduce others and be seduced is irresistible. Feelings of ease, intensity, power, well-being, financial omnipotence, and euphoria pervades one's very marrow. (Jamison 1995 cited in Wolpert 1999: 26–7)

Jamison goes on to describe a manic time when she bought books simply on the basis of the way a cover looked or a title sounded.

During one such book buying spree she purchased volumes on the natural history of the mole, and twenty books published by Penguin thinking it would be nice if the penguins on the covers could form a colony. However, although some aspects of this wildly euphoric condition might seem amusing, bipolar disorders remain personally and socially very debilitating. On the other hand, the creative, risk-taking element in the condition might account for the higher than expected number of sufferers who are in business, politics, the arts and the professions.

Anxiety Disorders

Emotional plans are a wonderful addition to emotional auto-maticity. They allow us to be emotional *actors* rather then just *reactors*. But the capacity to make this switch has a price. Once you start thinking, not only do you try to figure the best thing to do in the face of several possible next moves that a predator (including social predator) is likely to make, you also think about what will happen if the plan fails. Bigger brains allow better plans, but for these you pay in the currency of anxiety . . . (LeDoux 1996: 177)

Anxiety itself is a normal part of everyday life. Fear and anxiety can be adaptive responses to any situation which is ambiguous or uncertain, threatening or stressful, harmful or potentially dangerous. Anxiety, as a form of fear, provokes a cautious, avoidance response which in evolutionary terms promotes survival. However, there is a difference: 'anxiety comes from within us, fear from the outside world' (LeDoux 1998: 228). It is only when anxiety becomes chronic, pervasive and ill-focused that it reaches the status of a disorder.

Many people suffer anxiety disorders. They are one of the most common categories of mental health disorder. The disorders frequently are found in tandem with a range of physical health complaints and difficulties which often can't be explained by doctors and seem to defy physical treatment. Excessive anxiety, chronic worry and sometimes fear characterize this condition. Typical of individuals with these disorders is the misperception of things and people as threatening. Sufferers assume that situations will not work out well. They have a negative bias when appraising events and their outcome. The condition can trouble people for months and years.

Women are twice as likely as men to be diagnosed suffering an anxiety disorder. There is a genetic component that makes some people more at risk than others but environmental factors also need to be present (Williams et al 2005). People who are biologically inhibited, easily aroused and are biased towards more negative affect are at increased risk of anxiety. This biological vulnerability is negatively influenced if the individual (i) has grown up feeling that they have limited control over an unpredictable environment which reduces feelings of self-efficacy and makes them very wary of and anxious about new experiences; (ii) experiences caregiving which is either over-controlling, over-protective, rejecting or neglectful; (iii) has not enjoyed good peer relationships; and (iv) experiences stress.

For example, if a child grows up perceiving that they cannot control much of what happens to them, they will feel increasingly anxious and fearful, particularly when they meet new situations. This helplessness increases the risk of the adult developing an anxiety disorder and may well see the emergence of a range of dysfunctional defensive behaviours to try and deal with the perceived threat. These defensive reactions include many of the specific and social anxieties, and obsessive-compulsive behaviours described below.

Over-protective and anxious parents risk undermining their children's sense of being able to control and predict the world (Williams et al 2005). Over-protected and over-controlled children are denied opportunities of learning how to deal on their own with situations that make them feel anxious or stressed. Children who have not developed ways of dealing with fear, stress and anxiety are likely to feel helpless when, in future, life throws difficult challenges their way. Children who have had successful experiences of dealing with risk themselves are more resilient. They become 'steeled' to deal well with difficulty and set-back. Matters are particularly problematic when the source of fear and uncertainty is the unpredictable behaviour of a hostile or helpless parent. Children are left feeling fearful and helpless and some, particularly the biologically inhibited, will go on to develop anxiety disorders and avoidance strategies of one kind or another. Similarly, children who suffer parental rejection, harsh criticism and belittlement have their competence constantly undermined. These children, especially the easily aroused and inhibited ones, quickly lose confidence and grow increasingly anxious in new situations.

As we have seen, both fear and anxiety have adaptive value. In states of fear and panic, hearts beat faster, the body and hands sweat, eyes open wide with vigilant anxiety, and escape routes are desperately sought. Fear triggers flight responses, while feelings of anxiety make an individual wary and likely to avoid situations that make them feel nervous. So, in strict survival terms, fear is entirely functional. It invites a rapid flight-fight reaction in the face of sudden danger. It only becomes a problem when feelings of fear arise in objectively non-threatening situations including social situations, or when feelings of panic overwhelm someone without warning.

A threat creates a fast-track reaction in the amygdala and initially bypasses the cortex. Fear is felt before it is thought about. In the case of anxiety, matters are reversed. Thinking makes people feel anxious. Cognition and emotion are linked as the individual feels helpless and not able to control events. There is no immediate danger. The threat is an imagined possibility, and therein lies the anxiety. Vigilance is required in order to spot any potential signs of danger and distress. One must be prepared at all times and so the individual can never relax, even though the threat is vague and poorly defined. Apprehension and a general anxiety pervade both body and mind. A lot of mental and physical energy is therefore spent trying to ward off the anxiety. The result is worry and the avoidance of situations that might present the imagined danger. The individual's thought processes appear to be dominated by anticipated threats about which they imagine they can do little. In this way, negative thinking distorts the way situations are perceived and appraised.

These cognitive distortions tend to exaggerate threats, over-estimate danger, and downplay one's ability to do anything about them. 'Considerable evidence supports the existence of anxiety-related cognitive distortions and information-processing biases in both adult and child populations' (Williams et al 2005: 308). Appraisal is closely linked to the emotional centres of the brain, so if the evaluations are persistently negative then the predominant emotional state will also be negative and dominated by feelings of dread.

There are a variety of anxiety disorders. *Generalised Anxiety Disorder*, as the name suggests, occurs when there is a tendency to suffer pervasive worry over what appear to be relatively minor concerns. Stress levels tend to be high, and people experience relationship, work and health problems.

Perhaps one of the most familiar anxiety disorders is the diagnosis of a *specific phobia*. People may react to the feared thing or situation with feelings of panic, or they might faint. Their hearts pound. They sweat. What specific thing precipitates a feeling of panic and fear in the individual can be extremely varied. However, they seem to fall into five main categories, some of which from an evolutionary survival perspective seem more understandable than others given that some snakes and spiders can kill. People may suffer a fear of:

- some kind of animal (for example: snakes, spiders, moths);
- natural environments (for example: heights, water);
- blood (for example: injections, seeing blood);
- situations (for example: underground trains, enclosed spaces, crowded places, flying, lifts);
- anything else.

Social phobia is present when the individual experiences fear should they find themselves or think about finding themselves in a social situation where they imagine they would be under scrutiny. Social phobics are hypervigilant and ultra-sensitive to social situations in which they might be frightened, made anxious, rejected, feel a fool, shamed or ridiculed. The trigger can be as mild as simply being in a social group or meeting the opposite sex, or as severe as being asked to give a public lecture or lead a seminar. Clearly the former is the most debilitating type of *social anxiety* as it applies to most social situations, although it might exist in very particular forms such as fear of eating and drinking in public.

Panic disorder, perhaps known more familiarly as 'panic attack', involves a sudden, intense surge of fear in which the individual has a racing, palpitating heart; sweats; suffers chest pains; feels sick; feels dizzy; and fears they might die. There is an overwhelming urge to escape the situation. Once they are over the attack, people then worry about when it will happen again. Typical of people who suffer panic attacks is feeling panicky about the physiological affects of anxiety – heart palpitations, sweating, shaking, feeling faint – producing a feedback affect that leads to the full blown panic attack itself. They misinterpret the body's normal responses to stress believing that they are going to die or suffer some horrible catastrophe such a major heart attack.

Agoraphobia is experienced when individuals avoid getting into situations where they imagine they might have a panic attack but they will be unable to escape to a place of safety. A foreboding sense of potential helplessness prevents them venturing beyond the safe confines of home or putting themselves in any new kind of situation or environment (travelling on a bus, visiting a shopping mall). Unfortunately, for the majority of sufferers, panic attacks and agoraphobia tend to be not only debilitating but also long term.

Obsessive-Compulsive Disorder (OCD) witnesses individuals behaving obsessively and feeling compelled to carry out one or more behaviours before they can continue with the rest of their day. A woman might be fearfully obsessed with the thought that she might be contaminated by germs, so she has to wash her hands repeatedly until her hands bleed. All of this has to be done before she can finally leave the house, meet guests, prepare food, or leave the bathroom.

A man might not be able to settle until he has put all the cutlery in a very specific order of size and purpose. He has to check this order many times before he leaves the kitchen only to find that he feels compelled to straighten the curtains so that they meet exactly half way across the windows. He steps back to see whether they are symmetrically aligned but never feels entirely comfortable that he has achieved the perfect order he so anxiously desires. His days are dominated by this compulsive ordering, checking, returning, repeating to make sure a door is locked or the lights are turned off.

> Compulsions represent ritualized patterns of behaviour or cognition that the person feels driven to perform to reduce anxiety or distress associated with an obsession or to prevent some dreaded consequence from occurring . . . The most common compulsions include washing and cleaning, counting, checking, repeating actions, and ordering. (Williams et al 2005: 296)

Post Traumatic Stress Disorder (PTSD) is suffered by people who have experienced an extreme trauma, such as rape, a car crash, violent physical and sexual abuse, or intense enemy fire in a war-zone. Witnessing a violent, life threatening event can also lead to PTSD. A child who observes domestic violence or a passer-by who witnesses a murder might suffer PTSD. In the aftermath of the trauma, they develop a range of symptoms including (i) re-experiencing the trauma in the form of flashbacks and intrusive memories in which the original terror feels present and very real leaving the person shaking, agitated, sweating, and with a pounding heart; (ii) avoidance, numbing, detachment, dissociation, and hopelessness; and (iii) increased arousal so that any sudden stimulus or reminder of the original trauma causes an exaggerated startle response, irritability, anger, hypervigilance, and sleeping problems.

Childhood Behavioural Problems and Disorders

When children and adolescents behave in ways which the general community find antisocial, disruptive and troubling, we are describing a range of disorders familiar to most child welfare specialists. Conduct disorders, externalising behaviours, oppositional defiant disorders (ODD) and attention deficit/hyperactivity disorders (ADHD) all include excess displays of frustration, anger, and aggression, emotions that the child appears unable to regulate. However, although there is considerable overlap in the diagnoses of anti-social/aggressive behaviours and ADHD, the two disorders are separate and distinct. ADHD, as the term suggests, is mainly a problem of maintaining attention and displaying restless, exaggerated, fidgety, hyperactivated behaviour. Children wander off task very easily, talk incessantly and run around a lot, often in situation where it is not appropriate such as school. There is the suggestion that young children diagnosed with ADHD are at risk of developing ODD in the middle years and conduct disorders in later childhood (Lahey et al 2000). Underlying each of these disruptive disorders are a number of temperamental and cognitive vulnerabilities. These can manifest themselves in a range of problem behaviours whenever the child experiences a stressful environment, particularly a stressful social environment.

Conduct disorders include a range of anti-social behaviours: stealing, running away from home, burglary, starting fires, aggression, verbal abuse. In this sense, these disruptive behaviours represent the extreme end of a continuum of childhood and adolescent conduct and behavioural problems (Hankin et al 2005: 387). Children who develop antisocial behaviours find it difficult to recognize and interpret certain facial expressions in other people, particularly fear and sadness. This inability to emotionally resonate with others impairs their ability to be empathic.

Children who develop anti-social behaviours at very young ages are most at risk of becoming delinquent, criminal and aggressive in adolescence and on into adulthood. For example, Huesman et al (1984) found that eight year old children described as aggressive by their peers were more likely to show aggression, be violent and commit crime when they reached the age of thirty. In contrast, children who display problem behaviours for the first time in adolescence tend to grow out of them (Moffit 1993). Although relatively few in number, the early onset group of problem behaviour adolescents and adults tend to account for most of the anti-social and criminal behaviour in society. The majority of children and adolescents diagnosed with conduct disorders are male. However, this may reflect the way males and females manifest aggressive behaviour. Whereas boys tend to be directly and physically aggressive, girls are more likely to show indirect aggression including verbal assaults and relationship aggression.

Children who are biologically biased towards the more negative emotions (fractious, impulsive, irritable) and who score less well in cognitive and verbal tests appear most at risk of developing conduct disorders when they also live in stressful environments (poor parenting, abusive parenting, family conflict, poverty, poor housing, rundown and high crime neighbourhoods, anti-social peers, media portrayals of violence) (Loeber and Farrington 2000). Certain temperamental vulnerabilities also make it more likely that children living in stressful conditions will behave antisocially. As well as more negative emotional biases, children who are daring, sensation seekers and not naturally very pro-social, empathic or inclined to feel guilt might follow more delinquent developmental pathways. Rejection by prosocial peers is a common experience for this group of children. This denies them opportunities to develop social interactional skills and improve social cognition. As a result, they gravitate towards other anti-social peers.

As in most forms of psychopathology it is the interaction between vulnerability factors (genetics, temperament, negative emotional bias) and environmental stressors that increases the risk of children behaving in disruptive and antisocial ways. A particularly potent combination is the interaction between heritable traits associated with aggression and being raised by physically abusive parents in violent family households. *Genetically vulnerable* children reared in these *stressful environments* are at high risk of conduct disorders and pronounced anti-social behaviours (Caspi et al 2002, Foley 2004). Hankin and colleagues neatly knit together the various themes of this section to account for which children might be diagnosed as conduct disordered:

> Clearly, as stressors are experienced in environmental contexts, individuals with heightened emotional vulnerability (e.g., poor emotion-regulation skills as instantiated biologically with greater amygdala activity and lowered prefrontal cortex activity) are more likely to feel negative emotions (e.g., anger, frustration) more quickly, to experience a longer duration of such negative affect, and to take longer to return to an emotional baseline; as a result, such youth would be more likely to respond behaviourally with greater aggression and more behavioral problems. (Hankin et al 2005: 400)

The interaction between nature and nurture is therefore likely to be highly complex. Vicious circles can easily set in. A temperamentally difficult and aggressive child increases the chance of parents behaving in a hostile and critical manner which will fuel the child's temper, and so on. Thus, when negative temperament interacts with an adverse environment, a poor psychosocial outcome is more likely. The interplay between the two risk factors increases children's vulnerability to a range of emotional and behavioural disorders.

Thus, mothers and fathers who are high on criticism, low on warmth, and more likely to use physical chastisement have children at significantly increased risk of mental health and behavioural problems (Richman et al 1982). Only the most temperamentally resilient children or those removed and placed with highly sensitive substitute carers might escape abusive and neglectful childhoods relatively unscathed. This reminds us that protective factors can sometimes mitigate the worst effects of even the most adverse parenting or negative biological inheritance (for example, impaired cognitive ability or a negative temperament). Some well known protective factors include the availability of an alternative caring and protective adult (for example, a grandmother or aunt), or success and recognition at school. Protective factors improve children's resilience. Good self-esteem, self-efficacy, and emotional intelligence can help even the most disadvantaged children rise above their lot.

It was Rutter (1979) who observed that although any one risk might not increase the likelihood of a child developing a psychiatric disorder compared to children suffering no risk, the combination of two or more risks does raise the chances of children experiencing mental health problems. Indeed, children exposed to four or five of the known risks or stresses of parental depression, family conflict, abuse and neglect, loss and separation, poverty, large family size, and parental criminality have their chances of developing a psychiatric disorder increased twenty-fold. But although multiple risks certainly increase children's vulnerability to psychopathology, we can only fully understand a child's pathway through the life course when we also consider what protective factors have entered the developmental equation. Risk factors increase vulnerability. Protective factors raise resilience. It is the dynamic interplay between children's exposure to risk on the one hand and experiences of protection on the other that determine whether the balance tips a child towards increased resilience or vulnerability. Vulnerable children in high risk environments are at the greatest risk of developing anti-social behaviour.

Personality Disorders

The diagnostic label of Personality Disorder (PD) begs the question what is personality that we can recognize a disordered one when we see it. This is still a vexed question, but in general terms personality disorder describes cases in which an individual displays a personality trait that is rigid, lacks flexibility and is used invariantly and maladaptively in all situations. Personality Disordered individuals have major problems in conducting everyday relationships functionally and with social competence. Many people with the disorder do not recognize or understand the dysfunctional nature of their personality traits and emotional biases. They lack 'insight' and tend to blame others for the problems they create. Others might simply describe them as having a 'difficult personality'. Indeed, it can be the case that some Personality Disorders might allow the individual to fit well into a certain cultural environment or even flourish (Lemma 1996: 183). For example, obsessive traits might be valued by a company that demands high standards and attention to detail. Or people with narcissistic traits might perform larger than life on the stage or in the arts, lapping up the attention, love and admiration proffered by adoring fans.

PDs are not illnesses or medical conditions as such but clearly they create problems for individuals and those around them. There are many types of Personality Disorder including anti-social, dependent, narcissistic, paranoid and schizoid. They can be grouped into three main clusters (DSM-IV as cited by Lemma 1996: 180), although individual patients might be diagnosed with more than one type:

Cluster A: Paranoid, schizoid and schizotypal (typically characterized by 'eccentric' behaviours).

Cluster B: Antisocial, borderline, histrionic and narcissistic (typically characterized by impulsive and dramatic behaviour).

Cluster C: Avoidant, dependent and obsessive-compulsive (typically characterized by anxiety and fear).

Most people who are diagnosed with Personality Disorder (PD) describe childhoods in which they suffered adversity of one kind or another – abuse, neglect, parental loss, rejection. Certain combinations of physical abuse, emotional abuse, sexual abuse, emotional neglect and physical neglect increase the risk of particular types of PD. For example, combinations of childhood physical abuse and neglect generally increase the risk of developing Antisocial PD, whereas any kind of neglect on its own elevates the risk of Dependent PD (a personality pattern in which people seek dependency, fear abandonment, can't make decisions, behave in a clinging and submissive way).

We have seen in Chapter Five that childhood abuse, neglect and trauma adversely affect brain development and activity. However, this does not rule out possible genetic and prenatal factors playing a part. The interaction of genetic, prenatal vulnerability factors and parental maltreatment increases the risk of developing PDs (Caspi et al 2002, Foley et al 2004).

For example, it may be hypothesized that young children who have a relatively anxious, shy, or inhibited temperament may be especially like to develop a Cluster C (i.e., avoidant, dependent, obsessive-compulsive) PD if they are emotionally neglected during their formative years. Young children with an outgoing, gregarious temperament many be most likely to develop a Cluster B PD (i.e., antisocial, borderline, narcissistic, and histrionic PDs) if physically, sexually or emotionally abused. (Johnson et al 2005: 420)

Abuse and neglect cause repeated arousal and severe emotional dysregulation so that children find it difficult to understand and therefore manage their own and other people's affective states. This deficit upsets subsequent socialization experiences with parents, peers, and teachers denying children further opportunities to explore and modulate their own and other people's emotional arousal. The inability to regulate feelings and behave appropriately in the context of relationships broadly defines the Personality Disorders.

By way of illustration, we shall consider only two PDs, Antisocial Personality Disorder (ASPD) and Borderline Personality Disorder (BPD). ASPD, sometimes described as 'psychopathic personality', describes a person who is impulsive, aggressive, reckless, lawless, unpredictable, prone to boredom, superficially charming, callous, indifferent to the needs of others, and showing a total disregard for and violation of the rights of those with whom they interact. They lack remorse. Many people in the prison population are diagnosed with ASPD. Many have childhood histories of physical abuse, sexual abuse, neglect, and parental rejection. As children, many developed conduct disorders.

Carl witnessed much domestic violence as a child. When he was 13, his father killed his mother with a knife during an alcohol-fuelled argument. His father was sent to prison. Carl, who had a history of being excluded from school for violent behaviour, was placed in residential care. He took a range of drugs. On one occasion he caused a great deal of distress when he strangled one of the home's cats 'to see what it felt like to kill something'. He expressed no sorrow saying that 'it was old and smelled anyway'. Many of the other children in the home were frightened of him. When Carl was 17, he committed a violent robbery in which he cut the face of his victim 'to let him know I called. I only took what was in his wallet, so I don't know why everyone is so bothered'.

Many patients with Borderline Personality Disorder (BPD) report childhood physical abuse, sexual abuse, emotional abuse, emotional neglect and/or physical neglect. These early traumatic relational experiences, typically with parents and primary caregivers, affect brain development such that sufferers find it difficult to integrate cognition and emotion. They find it hard to think about feeling. They therefore find it very difficult to regulate their emotions. Their sense of self lacks coherence which means they can ricochet from one thought and feeling to another without any apparent pattern or predictability either to others or themselves.

People with BPD experience many emotions and violent mood swings at intense, unregulated and overwhelming levels, particularly in the context of relationships. They cannot tolerate anxiety and have to act immediately. Anger, hostility, anxiety, loneliness and depression can all be felt with some ferocity. They are afraid of being alone and yet when they are with people they are unable to regulate their feelings of love and hate. Parallel behaviours can include suicidal gestures, self-harm, avoidance, overreacting, aggression, destructive acts and impulsivity, perhaps as attempts to try and regulate these strong negative emotions (Kring and Werner 2004: 376). Feelings of emptiness cause despair and depression.

BPD sufferers can both idealize and denigrate other people, often the same person at different times. This leads to relationships in which the neediness at the heart of BPD leads to intense dependence and need of the other person one moment only to be followed by angry and contemptuous dismissal the next. The idealized and hostile evaluations are projections and not based on a realistic appraisal of the other person. The result is relationships that are conflict ridden. Individuals with BPD have been found to be relatively unaware, and certainly unable to reflect on their own and other people's emotional condition. As a result, they show little empathy. Not being aware of their own emotional displays and how they impact on others, they are unable to regulate their arousal. This leads to dramatic, out-of-control displays of most of the negative emotions.

> Emma, the parent of two young girls, had been having a series of short-lived, conflict-ridden relationships which had quickly broken down. For the last four weeks she had been dating Rick.

Their affair had been intense as they spent nearly every moment together. Emma said she loved him passionately and had planned the names of the children they were going to have together. However, she began to feel that Rick was cooling off. She demanded his commitment but he responded equivocally. Her response was first to self-harm by cutting her arms with a razor blade and then on an impulse she swallowed 25 of her sedatives. Emma was found unconscious by a neighbour who had collected the girls from nursery. Emma was rushed to hospital. Rick paid a fleeting visit to her while she was in hospital but they got into an argument almost immediately. He walked out. She told the social worker that she hated him, that no-one loved her, and she didn't want to live any more. It was after this incident that Emma began to visit the social worker almost daily telling her that she was the first person to really understand her. But when the social worker was away on a week's training course, Emma smashed the glass of the reception office shouting that 'no fucker gave a toss about her, least of all that bitch who called herself a social worker'. As there were child care concerns, the relationship with the worker continued but was characterised by emotional turbulence, apologies by Emma, followed by virulent criticism, expressions of pain and rejection.

Dementia

Emotions and our characteristic ways of expressing them are so tied up with our personalities and how others view us that it can come as something of a sad shock to relatives of some older people to realize that the degenerative diseases that attack the brain and destroy neurons on a massive scale change both our personalities and the kind of emotional beings we are. Although the body of the sufferer stays the same, the mind, and hence the person are no longer quite as they were.

The particular emotional changes affecting an individual depend on which particular part of the brain and neurological structures are damaged. So, although emotional symptoms are common in dementia, the emotional changes wrought by the disease might vary in detail between individuals. Apathy and indifference can affect some. Anxiety and fretful worry over nothing in particular can bother others. It is not at all unusual for some people to become tearful and even depressed. Others giggle for no apparent reason. Disinhibition is also a feature in some cases. Individuals act impulsively and inappropriately without embarrassment. And irritability and displays of bad temper, even aggression can be characteristic.

The distressing aspect of these changes in emotional behaviour for relatives is that they are out of character with the person they have known and lived with for so many years. The previously mild mannered mother becomes impatient and quick of temper. The husband known for his quiet stoicism now cries easily and wanders around the house looking agitated and confused.

Although most dementias involve some behavioural and emotional disorder, the exact character of the disorder depends on which area of the brain is undergoing degeneration. Semantic dementia (associated with language disorder) and Alzheimer's Disease both involve some disturbance of the emotions including increased apathy, anxiety, irritability, depression and agitation.

Other types of dementia seem to affect the limbic system including the front temporal lobes, amygdala and prefrontal cortex. As we saw in Chapter Five, these parts of the brain are involved in the experience of emotions and their regulation, and therefore social behaviour. Patients who suffer this particular form of dementia (frontotemporal lobar dementia or FTLD) suffer emotional blunting, lack of empathy and insight, and low motivation (Rosen et al 2002). Emotional cues that oil the wheels of relationships are no longer recognized or understood. The more self-conscious social emotions of embarrassment, guilt, pride and shame seem particularly affected, although the basic emotions such as fear associated with the amygdala seem unaffected. And interestingly, with these emotional losses, facial expressions reduce and emotional vocabulary diminishes. Sufferers find it difficult to suppress their feelings and so begin to behave in ways that family and friends feel are inappropriate and uncharacteristic. They can be rude, crude and in some cases aggressive. Social interaction becomes difficult. Carers and families can find these behaviours difficult to manage. To close relatives it feels as if the sufferer has had a change of personality, and in the sense that key areas of the emotional brain are being destroyed this would be true.

Conclusion

Emotions in excess or deficit characterize many mental health concerns and behavioural problems. It is a strong reminder that the ability to regulate emotions and empathize with others is one of the defining qualities of social competence. Without this kind of emotional intelligence social life becomes very difficult. Relationships are put under strain and liable to break down.

One of the major downsides of emotionally under-regulated and over-regulated behaviour is the social opprobrium and isolation that individuals suffer. Cut off from the pleasure of smooth running relationships and easy social acceptance, people whose emotions are out of balance face further stress. Their behaviour denies them the benefits of learning from others about the value of emotions and the intelligence that emotional awareness gives those who are comfortable acknowledging, exploring and reflecting on their own and other people's feelings. Over the next two chapters, we shall consider a number of therapies whose aim is to treat these emotional blind spots and the mental health and behavioural problems they create.

8
Cognitive and Behavioural Therapies

Introduction

Throughout many of the clinical and psychologically based professions, cognitive and behavioural therapies (CBT) are the treatment of choice. This is in part because they have chosen to go down the science route of evidence-based practice, and partly because this route has shown that for many mental health and behavioural problems CBT is effective. The rigour implied in these therapies has also proved attractive to other people-oriented professions that have been keen to show their relevance and effectiveness in areas of human behaviour in which it has been notoriously difficult to bring about change. In particular, probation officers, youth justice workers, and many social workers specialising in the mental health field have shown considerable interest in cognitive and behaviourally based treatment programmes.

In this chapter we shall concentrate on those cognitive and behavioural treatments that deal squarely with individuals experiencing severe dysfunction and dysregulation in their emotional lives.

Thought, Feeling and Behaviour

We might begin by reminding ourselves that emotions are processed and managed by many parts of the brain including the limbic system and cortex. This gives us a clue about why different kinds of treatment and support might be equally effective in helping people who are finding it difficult to regulate their arousal or interact with others in an emotionally skilled fashion. Different therapies are addressing different parts of our neurological and emotional development, make-up and functioning.

The aim of most therapies is to help the individual (and their brains) make links between their thoughts, feelings and behaviours so that they become more aware of the complexities of their own psychological functioning. If this process is successful, the patient or service user recovers control over his or her own experience and behaviour.

> When memories are stored in sensory and emotional networks but are dissociated from those that organize cognition, knowledge, and perspective, we become vulnerable to intrusions of past experiences that are triggered by environmental and internal cues. In the process of psychotherapy, we attempt to reintegrate these dissociated networks by conscious cortical processing to develop the ability to inhibit and control past traumatic memories. (Cozolino 2006: 32)

Cognitive processes play a key role in helping us to read, manage and reflect on our own and other people's feelings. It is therefore likely that cognitive-based therapies will be relevant when dealing with certain types of emotional problem. We have also learned that feeling that you have little control over your environment, that it seems unpredictable, is stressful, and that stress leads to anxiety. Achieving a sense of control also requires that thought takes charge of negative feeling, and so cognitive-based treatments are likely to be of value here too.

The second therapeutic approach seeks its inspiration from the way children develop emotional understanding and intelligence. Affect regulation, theory of mind and empathy develop as young minds relate and engage with emotionally attuned and sensitive older minds. When we interact with someone who is willing and able to understand us at the emotional level, we receive valuable information about our own affective make-up. This 'making sense' of our own emotional being is reflected in the growing complexity, coherence and integrity of our brains and the psychological self it supports. Emotion and cognition are linked at both the neurological and psychological level. The thought centres of the brain get into rich communication with the feeling centres.

In secure relationships with an empathic other, we feel safe to explore our feelings. If we feel contained and understood, it becomes possible to think about feeling. If we have never learned to regulate our arousal, when our only experience is that feelings overwhelm us and make us angry or sad or ashamed or anxious, then emotions are something to fear. Our emotions have a habit of quickly getting out-of-control. This is frightening. We may try to avoid our hurts and fears through drink or drugs. We may feel increasing despair as we lose grip on our own destiny. It is the aim of the more humanistic and developmental psychotherapies to offer a relationship in which many of the features of high-quality parent–child interactions are present. Emotional attunement, affective mirroring, affect recognition, containment and empathy help individuals learn to regulate their own arousal.

Person-centred approaches, attachment-based therapies, psychodynamic therapies, group work, social support and community development in part seek to build up people's self-esteem, reflective capacities and emotional intelligence. They mimic many of the features that characterise emotionally intelligent parenting.

The purpose of this chapter and the next is not to provide a full account of each therapeutic school's theory and practice. Rather it is to give a sense of how different therapies try to help people make sense of their own and other people's emotions and ultimately gain control over their own affective states. Following the idea that the brain is a complex neurological structure in which emotions are processed, managed and expressed cognitively, behaviourally and interpersonally, we shall consider supports and interventions that are based on one or more of the following premises:

- Helping people change their *behaviour vis-à-vis* an emotionally inducing event will result in a change of emotional experience – change the behaviour and you change the feeling (behaviour therapy).
- Helping people change their *thinking* (or *cognitions*) *vis-à-vis* an emotionally inducing event will result in changes of emotional experience – change the thinking and you change the feeling (cognitive therapy).
- Helping people *develop emotional understanding* and affect regulation in the context of an empathic, attuned relationship will improve their emotional intelligence (relationship-based therapies).

Behavioural and cognitive based interventions are the focus of the present chapter. Relationship-based supports and treatments are considered in the next.

Behaviour Therapy

Scientists in the behavioural tradition are interested in how behaviours are acquired and how they are maintained (or lost). Their work has produced a range of treatments, many of which seem particularly effective in helping people troubled by high levels of the more negative emotions including fear, anxiety and anger.

It was Watson and Raynor (1920), developing Pavlov's original research, who discovered that if an emotional reaction could be learned then it could be unlearned. The learning and unlearning are achieved by a process known as *classical conditioning* or 'respondent conditioning'. It is the basis of a number of behavioural therapies.

Pavlov, of course, was famous for teaching dogs to salivate at the sound of a bell. He observed that dogs naturally salivate when given meat (or in his case meat powder). After a while he also noticed that the dogs actually began to salivate as their handlers approached in preparation to feeding the dogs. In order to test this association, Pavlov experimented with the dogs as follows.

Prior to the experiment, the sound of a bell ringing would not cause the dogs to salivate. So, in the first part of the experiment, just before the dogs were about to be fed, a bell or tuning fork would ring. The dogs therefore began to associate the ringing of the bell with the arrival of food. It was only a matter of time before the bell ringing on its own, without the presentation of food, would cause the dogs to salivate. Pavlov had brought about a new response that was not there before. Salivation could now be triggered by the bell alone.

More technically, what had happened was that an 'unconditioned stimulus' (UCS) – in this case food – automatically or naturally produced an 'unconditioned response' (UCR) – salivation. Next, a 'conditioned stimulus' – the bell – was introduced prior or simultaneously to the appearance of the food. In time, a response conditional on the appearance of the new stimulus is achieved, that is a conditioned stimulus (CS) – the bell – brings about a 'conditional response' (CR) – salivation.

Behaviourists believe that many phobias are acquired through a similar process of conditioning. In what may now appear to be a rather ethically unsound experiment, Watson and Raynor (1920), showed how a fear or phobia could develop. The unlucky subject was eleven month old Little Albert. Before the conditioning, Little Albert showed no natural fear of either rats or rabbits. Watson and Raynor then introduced a conditioned stimulus whenever Little Albert was presented with a tame rat. They clanged a steel bar with a hammer producing a frighteningly loud noise that startled Little Albert as he quietly watched the rat. It was only a matter of time before Little Albert simply had to see a rat on its own, with no loud clang, for him to become distressed. This fear of rats, induced by the alarming noise, soon began to 'generalize' to a fear of all furry objects including rabbits. We are never told what happened to Little Albert, whether or not the adult Albert was equally terrified whenever he saw a rat, rabbit or fur coat.

However, in kinder hands, it became apparent that classical conditioning could be used therapeutically. If a pleasurable stimulus could be associated with an existing unconditioned fear response, say a fear of spiders, then maybe the fear could be extinguished. Wolpe (1990) developed this insight into a therapeutic procedure that we now know as *systematic desensitisation*, the treatment of choice for many phobias. Fears, he claimed, could be unlearned.

The treatment has three stages: (i) relaxation training, (ii) construction of a fear hierarchy, and (iii) a new learning process. Anxiety and fear are incompatible with pleasure and feeling relaxed. In treatment, the strength of the pleasure must outweigh the strength of the anxiety. The candidate is first taught to relax using a variety of techniques that best suit the individual. The next stage requires the patient to construct a hierarchy of fear in which the most feared situation is scored at say a 100 per cent while things that cause no anxiety whatsoever are rated at 0 per cent, with a number of situations and their ratings placed in between the lowest and highest.

A person with agoraphobia may be able to answer a knock at the door (fear rating = 0 per cent), but experiences mild distress when they walk to the garden gate. The idea of journeying to the end of the street is more fearful while the thought of being in a busy shopping mall induces feelings of total panic (fear rating = 100 per cent). The patient is first asked to imagine strolling to the garden gate while practising the relaxation technique. This is repeated until the thought of being at the gate causes no anxiety. So what was say a 5 per cent anxiety level is now the new zero level. The next stage up in the original fear hierarchy is next 'visited' using the same technique, until finally the previously most feared situation, the shopping mall, can be contemplated without anxiety.

Some therapists will actually ask the patient to progress through each stage for real, not as an imagined exercise but *in vivo*. In the case of the agoraphobic patient, as well as practising relaxation techniques, a friend or reassuring therapist might initially accompany the individual as they negotiate each level of the fear hierarchy. The increasing feeling of confidence and control in situations that used to cause anxiety acts as a further pleasurable stimulus. Along similar lines, Hudson and Macdonald (1986: 122) give the example of treating a school phobic. The child is gradually exposed, and then desensitised to situations that originally caused varying degrees of distress:

1. Walking past school (with social worker, then alone).
2. Standing outside school at weekend (with social worker, then alone).
3. In school with social worker at weekend.
4. In classroom with teacher at weekends.
5. In playground with social worker on a school day.
6. In school building on a school day but not in class.
7. In school, in class with other children.

Phobias can seriously disrupt people's lives. A mother with agoraphobia might begin to rely more and more on her young daughter to shop and run errands. As a result the young girl's school work and friendships begin to suffer. A man who develops a fear of running water might find his journey to work becoming virtually impossible as he devises more and more tortuous routes to avoid any risk of passing a stream, a brook, a burst water main, or a street gutter on a rainy day.

We have seen that classical conditioning examines how a stimulus can produce a *new behaviour*. However, the process that looks at how an *existing behaviour* can be increased in frequency, duration or intensity is known as *operant conditioning* (or 'instrumental conditioning'). It was Thorndike who found that if a behaviour leads to a positive or desired outcome, it is likely to be repeated in similar situations in the future. If a behaviour produces a negative or unpleasant outcome, it is less likely that it will be repeated in similar situations. So, if every time a dog is rewarded with a biscuit when it comes to heel at the sound of whistle, it will not be long before the dog responds in the desired way each time the whistle is blown. Skinner developed Thorndike's ideas and termed any environmental response that increased a behaviour a *reinforcer* and any environmental response that decreased the occurrence of a behaviour a *punishment*.

Thus, whereas in classical conditioning the environment (the appearance of a snake) causes a behavioural reaction (fear), matters are reversed in operant conditioning. The behaviour (coming to heel at the sound of a whistle) 'causes' the environment to respond (a rewarding dog biscuit appears). The biscuit acts as a *positive reinforcement*. The individual's behaviour, in effect, 'operates' on the environment triggering a response (either a reward or punishment).

According to behavioural psychologists, many of the undesired behaviours shown by children (for example, excessive temper tantrums, frequent aggression, persistent food refusal) have actually been made worse by parents unwittingly reinforcing their occurrence. When a child gets frustrated with a task and gets angry, the parent intervenes, even if the intervention is a verbal telling off. However, when the child is playing happily without any upset, the parent ignores him, goes into the kitchen or sneaks off to the local shop. From the child's point of view, any parental recognition, acknowledgement or interest is better than none. Attention nearly always acts as a reinforcer. If the parent supplies recognition, acknowledgement or interest only when the child misbehaves, in effect they are reinforcing 'angry and difficult behaviour' and punishing positive, task-achieving, constructive play behaviour by ignoring it. Similarly, if a toddler screams and a bag of crisps is thrown her way or a TV is switched on, screaming behaviour is reinforced. As a result, yelling becomes an ever more likely response whenever needs are felt.

It is also possible to *increase* behaviours by *removing an aversive stimuli* or unpleasant response. This is known as a *negative reinforcement* (which is not to be confused with punishment). For example, if traffic wardens are removed from the streets, there is a likely to be an increase in illegal parking.

Punishments are environmental responses that lead to a *decrease* in a behaviour. *Positive punishments* involve the *introduction of an aversive response*. Pocket money is stopped if a child is aggressively rude to parents in the hope that the obstreperous behaviour ceases. *Negative punishment* describes the *removal of a response that decreases a behaviour*.

For example, if a teacher stops praising a child who persists with a difficult task, the child might give up trying.

Simply *ignoring a behaviour* can also lead to its decline or *extinction*. In cases in which a parent is complaining of a child's difficult, unruly behaviour, a relatively simply behaviour modification programme might involve advising the parent to ignore the child's display of bad behaviour (extinction procedure) and reinforce examples of good, desired behaviour with praise, encouragement, and admiration (positive reinforcement procedures). Punishment procedures are rarely advised and can often be counter-productive.

Behavioural techniques first require a careful assessment of the problem: specify exactly what happens and who behaves in what manner before, during and after the emission of the undesired behaviour (ABC: antecedents – behaviour – consequences). Observations are made and questions asked about the frequency, duration, and intensity of the behaviour. By re-shaping the way the (social) environment reacts to behaviours, the aim is to decrease conduct that is problematic and increase behaviours that are desired.

In practice, these programmes tend to be more elaborate and sophisticated than outlined above, and often include other behavioural techniques such as role modelling and social skills training. They have been found to work well for children with oppositional defiant disorders (ODD) and conduct disorders (CD). In most cases, parents are advised to encourage prosocial behaviours and ignore disruptive behaviours. Parents are asked to be consistent and predictable in the way they react to both desired and undesired behaviour. For example, the Oregon Learning Center Programs (Patterson 1976; Eyberg et al 1995) typically work with children between the ages of 3 and 12 years. They focus on aggression and non-compliance. Parents are encouraged to observe their children's behaviour, note what happens before and after both positive and negative behavioural episodes, and then try out some positive reinforcement (particularly social attention and praise) and extinction procedures (ignoring bad behaviours). The programmes also include helping parents learn to problem solve and develop negotiation skills and strategies (also see the Forehand and McMahon (1981) program, and the Webster-Stratton (1999) program designed for teachers and parents of children with educational, behavioural and emotional needs).

Most behaviourally based interventions actually combine classical and operant conditioning techniques. Mowrer's (1947) 'two-factor' model recognized that in most situations a behaviour may well be acquired in the first place through classical conditioning, but it is then maintained through operant conditioning. For example, a person may have become frightened of aggressive dogs after a traumatic incident in which he was attacked by a pit bull terrier (factor one, classical conditioning). However, thereafter the mere avoidance of any dog keeps the man calm which positively reinforces 'keeping away from dogs' behaviour (factor two). When working with patients, behaviour therapists will assess and then treat the problem with both factors in mind.

Cognitive Therapies

If the heyday of behavioural psychology was the first half of the 20th century, then the second half witnessed the growing importance of cognitive psychology, the goal of which is to understand the working of human intelligence and the way we experience and process information. Human beings are defined as 'information processors'. Cognitive psychology covers such things as perception, attention, the way we mentally represent the world (including our selves) in our heads, memory, reasoning, problem-solving, language, and comprehension. It will be apparent from this list that whereas behavioural psychology concentrates on what can be directly observed, that is our behaviour, cognitive psychology is much more interested in what we see and think and why we see and think it.

Thought, of course, is a very powerful asset, but it can cause us trouble. Human beings have a tendency to think about all sorts of things, real and imagined, in the past and in the future, about themselves and other people. Within this mix there is considerable scope for misperception, misrepresentation and misunderstanding. And this is when thought processes can get distorted causing our mental experiences, and hence our feelings, to go awry. '[T]here is nothing either good or bad' said Shakespeare's Hamlet (Act II, Scene ii), 'but thinking makes it so'.

Cognitive therapists recognize that the way we think affects the way we feel. Our moods are deeply affected by our memories, assumptions, beliefs, perceptions and reasoning. People suffering mental health problems in which negative emotions predominate are thought to have a negative bias in the way they perceive and interpret events. Things are liable to be interpreted in the worst possible light leading to anxiety, depression or anger. The goal of cognitive therapy, therefore, is to change this negative bias in which perception and interpretation are cast most darkly. As with behavioural therapy, the basic principles are simple, but treatment practice in the hands of the most skilful and creative therapists is endlessly varied.

Ellis pioneered cognitive treatments in the 1950s but it was Beck whose refinements throughout the 1970s led to their present day success. Ellis (1962) proposed that problem behaviours and emotional distress are the result of irrational beliefs held about the self, others and situations. For example, people who believe that everything that they do must be done to perfection give themselves a difficult, if not impossible task. When they don't manage to behave or perform perfectly, they are at high risk of feeling a failure and becoming depressed. Or someone who believes that everyone should be loved and valued but doesn't feel loved or valued themselves, such a person might begin to feel increasingly anxious and distressed about their own perceived unlovability and worthlessness.

The task of the therapist is to help the individual change their beliefs to ones that are more reasonable and realistic. So rather than believe that you should be loved and liked by everyone, Joseph (2001: 104) gives the example that it is better to believe that 'It's good to be liked, but I can't expect everyone to appreciate me in the same way. Some people might not like me and that's OK: it's not essential for me that everyone likes me.' Ellis argues that the therapist must challenge, in a disputatious manner, the patient's irrational beliefs and then provide help to change them to a more rational set.

Beck also felt that negative ways of thinking that affect mood are illogical. In these mind-sets, people quickly magnify difficulties or read the wrong things into a situation. They seem to down play and ignore successes. As a result, their passive, fatalistic and negative views of people and events overwhelm them with feelings of depression and anxiety, even though objectively there is no evidence to support their outlook. Cited in Joseph (2001: 106–8), Beck and Weishaar (1989) note five steps in cognitive therapy:

1. Learning to monitor negative, automatic thoughts.
2. Learning to recognise the connection between cognition, affect and behaviour (that is how thought affects feeling and feeling affects behaviour).
3. Examining the evidence for and against distorted automatic thoughts.
4. Substituting more reality-oriented interpretations for these biased cognitions.
5. Learning to identify and alter the beliefs that predispose a person to distort their experiences.

Beck differs from Ellis in being less confrontational and more collaborative with the patient. The conceptual underpinnings of cognitive therapy are explained to the client and illustrated. Clients are first asked to try and become aware, name and then fully describe their negative feelings. This helps them connect with their inner emotional selves. For example, Wolpert, whom we first met in the previous chapter, reflecting on his own treatment for depression writes 'if the patient felt low and without hope before the session, the therapist would ask what thoughts were associated with these feelings. This can be used to illustrate the relationship between negative thoughts and feelings' (Wolpert 1999: 147–8). Problems are examined together by the therapist and patient. The dialogue is more Socratic in the sense that the therapist explores and examines what the patient is saying and the rational strength of the basis on which it is being said.

With the basic principles in mind, therapist and patient jointly work out ways to change and move forward. The patient is asked to review each session and say what conclusions they have drawn and understandings they have reached. Negative automatic ways of thinking about the self and situations are questioned. New, more positive ways of thinking about the previously negative mood inducing situation are discussed, rehearsed and tried.

Beck's cognitive therapies have been particularly successful in the treatment of depression and many of the anxiety disorders (Beck and Emery 1985). Depressed people tend to think negatively about the self, the world and the future. Negative memories are selectively recalled. The therapist seeks to alter these negative thinking patterns. Patients are taught to monitor and recognize whenever they find themselves slipping into Automatic Negative Thoughts (ANTs). The therapist will ask the patient to test the validity of the negative thought. The patient may say they have achieved nothing in life, or that no-one could care less about them. Upon examination such extreme negative thoughts tend to be exaggerated and rarely stand up to close scrutiny. It is these negative memories that are too readily brought to bear on current situations. Patients are then invited to consider if there might not be another, less gloomy way of thinking about the claim or situation. Techniques are introduced that are designed to help the patient not to activate old, bleak, negative memories.

A helpful book of case studies by Gorenstein and Comer (2002: 54) gives an example of the Socractic dialogue used by a cognitive therapist in the treatment of depression. Here is an extract of typical dialogue:

Dr. Waldon:	You say you are a 'basket case' and can barely function. What leads you to those conclusions?
Carlos:	Well, I've been hospitalized. That's how bad it's been. I just can't believe it . . . I told Dr Hsu my family might be better off without me.
Dr. Waldon:	Do you think they would be better off?
Carlos:	I don't know. I'm not doing them much good.
Dr. Waldon:	What would life be like for them without you?
Carlos:	It would be terrible for them. I suppose saying that they'd be better off without me is going too far. As bad off as I am, I'm still able to do a few things.
Dr. Waldon:	What are you able to do? . . .
Carlos:	I can't work, I can't help out at home, I can't even watch a television show . . .
Dr. Waldon:	A couple of minutes ago you said you were still able to do a few things. What are those?
Carlos:	I can drive to work and . . . I guess it's an exaggeration to say that I can't work at all. There are a few things I can do at the office.
Dr. Walden:	Like what?

And so on. By gently querying each negative thought, the therapist is seeking to dismantle the tendency automatically to go down the line of most negative thinking. Blackburn and Davidson's (1995) book on treating depression and anxiety also offers many examples of thera-pist-patient dialogue to illustrate dealing with automatic negative thoughts, mental imagery, examination of the evidence for the valid-ity of a thought, and the introduction of alternative interpretations when a negative spin has been given to an experience.

Other techniques are also used to bolster treatment. The use of mental imagery, role playing and diary keeping have all been shown to help. A course of cognitive therapy is structured, and relatively brief typically involving around 20 sessions over several months.

Cognitive Behavioural Therapies (CBT)

The combination of behavioural and cognitive therapies is the preferred method of treatment of many mental health specialists. Although behaviourally-based therapies have a longer pedigree than cognitive approaches, the two treatments began to join forces throughout the second half of the 20th century. Both aspire to be scientific and evidence-based in their approach. In terms of dealing with emotional dysregulation and the affective disorders, behav-ioural and cognitive therapies have been particularly effective in treating problems of mood such as depression, anxiety disorders including phobias, and conduct disorders. It is their combined effect that has proved so attractive to clinical psychologists, social workers, social care workers, probation officers, youth justice workers, and counsellors. Challenging irrational beliefs and automatic negative thinking are coupled with reinforcement procedures to encourage more positive behaviours. Helping people develop new, more up-beat activities helps people develop a more positive outlook.

For example, practitioners charged with mending the ways of youth and adult offenders have developed a range of service responses and treatment programmes heavily influenced by CBT. Not surprisingly, the emphasis by those working in prisons and in community-based probation and youth justice programmes tends to be on helping individuals stop committing crimes. The treatment focus is on encouraging offenders to think before they act (for a useful review of the efficacy of these offending behaviour programmes, see Roberts 2004). To the extent that poor emotional self-control might be a factor in triggering offending behaviour, emotions might or might not be directly addressed. For example, 'aggression replacement training programmes' offer offenders a multi-modal approach combining social skills training, self control training, and training in moral reasoning.

Psychologically and Medically-Based Treatments

It is also the case that some of the most effective CBT-based treatments work in tandem with drug medication. Not surprisingly, drugs that alter mood are used extensively to treat affective disorders. They act directly on the brain and so bring about changes of neurological and neurotransmitter functioning. For example, some psychoactive drugs act as anti-depressants by increasing or blocking a range of neurotransmitters. We have mentioned Prozac, but the drug Seroxat also increases levels of serotonin and noradrenaline in the brain and so helps reduce feelings of depression (see Chapter Five).

Anxiety disorders are commonly treated with sedatives such as the benzodiazepines which include Librium and Valium (diazepam). Patients who suffer bipolar disorder might be given a mood stabilizer (for example, Lithium).

Nearly all the psychoactive drugs have side effects, and some can become addictive. If CBT is to be combined with medication, careful monitoring and evaluation of the effects of the drug form an important part of the patient's management.

Conclusion

The strong evidence-based underpinnings of behavioural, cognitive and pharmacological treatments has made them particularly attractive to the more science-oriented professions, including psychiatry and clinical psychology. Nevertheless, many social workers have been influenced by and attracted to cognitive behaviour therapies, particularly those working in the fields of mental health, education, and anti-social and offending behaviour. Although it is often more difficult to design good research trials when testing the effectiveness of social work interventions, there is a growing willingness in some quarters to conceive, evaluate and promote practices that lend themselves to scientific scrutiny (for example, for a review of the effectiveness of interventions in probation and youth justice work, see

Burnett and Roberts 2004). Cognitive, behavioural, problem-solving and solution-seeking approaches have generally been more than happy to place themselves under the evidence-based microscope. However, most cognitive behavioural therapists also acknowledge the importance of the part that the relationship plays in the success of their treatments.

9
Relationship-Based Interventions and Social Support

Introduction

It has been argued that children learn about their own and other people's emotions and how to regulate them in the context of relationships – with parents, family, peers. Failures and problems with emotional recognition, understanding, containment and regulation develop when these primary relationships are with people who are insensitive, lack empathy, have no attunement, and cause distress and disturbance. It therefore follows that those who experience problems recognizing, experiencing and regulating their emotions are likely to benefit from forming relationships with people who are emotionally available and responsive, intelligent and psychologically-minded. If poor relationships are where things emotionally go wrong then healthy relationships are where things can be put right.

Behind this rather simple injunction lies a substantial body of theoretical, empirical and clinical support. Although it has been most clearly articulated within the psychoanalytic and psychodynamic traditions, valuable contributions and insights can be found in the broader humanistic-based therapies including person-centred approaches. This chapter will not attempt to do justice to the richness and depth of these various therapeutic approaches, rather it will follow those lines of thought that have linked relationships and emotional development (for a review, see Orlinsky and Howard 1986; Orlinsky et al 2004).

Making Links

Common to most therapies but particularly important in relationship-based help is the need for the practitioner to establish trust and a feeling of safety. Within the holding relationship service users feel safe enough to explore their feelings. In fact, if work and progress is to be made, users must experience some arousal and strength of feeling, whether the feelings are ones of anger, anxiety, shame, sadness, fear, or contempt. If the feelings can be felt, they become material on which to work, think about and reflect. Feelings that previously were unconscious but nevertheless were affecting behaviour and relationships in a powerful and often disruptive way can be brought to mind. This helps service users integrate thought and feeling, cognition and emotion.

Slowly, memories, relationship experiences, feelings, and behaviours can be linked. A narrative emerges. A story forms that begins to connect people and events, relationships and behaviour, feelings and defences, causes and effects. Stories intrigue us. They help us explore people's intention and motives. We want to know what happens next. We ask the question *why* in order to understand the psychological state and intent of the characters. Stories help us understand how the world of human affairs works.

It is when thought and feeling become more integrated, service users become better able to regulate their emotions. Making sense, and managing one's own and other people's feelings allows individuals to feel more in control. Making sense and feeling in control reduce anxiety and stress, and in their turn improve physical health and mental wellbeing.

Intersubjectivity and Psychotherapeutic Moments

Stern (2004) explores the therapeutic relationship at the level of 'minds meeting minds' in which some of our most profound experiences happen in key, meaningful moments. It is not even necessary for words to be present or exchanged for these moments to be experienced as significant. Both parties just 'know'. He describes these meetings of minds as the experience of *intersubjectivity*, a concept that we met in Chapter Four when we were considering mother–infant interaction and its importance in psychobiological regulation and the formation of the psychological self.

Intersubjectivity can be experienced during psychotherapy, or between close friends, or when we are in love. Stern believes that human beings seek out such connections. We need to understand

and be understood by others. In this sense, intersubjectivity is a basic motivational system that is as essential to survival as attachment or sex (Stern 2004: xvi). Intersubjectivity promotes group formation and cohesion. It facilitates co-operation. It allows us to be empathic and moral.

In moments of intersubjective connectedness we have the potential to be known by the other. Patients, clients and service users want to be known and understood. At some level, we are all desperate for other people to sense what it feels like to be us, even though to be understood can also make us feel vulnerable and frightened, hence our hesitancy and tentativeness and the need for trust before we can reach out to others. It is well for social workers to realize that even their most difficult service users at some level want to connect and be known. This might include recognizing and understanding their anger, fear, isolation, pain, desperation or sadness. To be recognized in the eyes of the other is to be helped to define and re-define, form and re-form the self (Stern 2004: 152).

In moments of heightened intersubjectivity we become conscious of our own mind and all its ineffable content as we feel recognized, understood and reflected by the other and the content of their mind. 'Two people', writes Stern (2004: 75), 'see and feel roughly the same mental landscape for a moment at least. These meetings are what psychotherapy is largely about.' These are rare, precious moments in which we experience our selves in a new, different, deepened and revealed manner. In the process, in the moment, in the 'here and now', we are changed. We move forward. Therapy, help and support are about such moments. Within them so much of who and what we are, and could be is revealed.

Stern quotes William Blake's line 'to see a world in a grain of sand' to capture the idea that so much of our personality, temperament, style and concerns can be revealed in such fleeting intersubjective moments. Besides being poetic, it captures:

> the size of the small world revealed by micro-analysis and at the same time [draws] attention to the fact that one can often see the larger panorama of someone's past and current life in the small behaviours and mental acts making up this micro-world. (Stern 2004: xiv)

The therapist, social worker, probation officer, counsellor or support worker must try and stay with the service user at these deeper, affective psychosubjective levels. The momentary surges and fades of feeling that we have second by second in any relationship can tell us much about ourselves if we can manage to stop, recognize, acknowledge and reflect. Why the sudden irritation? Where did that come from? Why the flash of anxiety and our immediate defensive reaction? What are its origins and effects? Much of this intersubjective resonance takes place outside spoken language. We feel the other's facial expressions, read their body language. We 'mind-read'. Our very social nature as a species means that:

> Our nervous systems are constructed to be captured by the nervous systems of others, so that we can experience others *as if* from within their skin, as well as from within our own. A sort of direct feeling route into the other person is potentially open and we resonate with and participate in their experiences, and they in ours. (Stern 2004: 76)

When motivated to experience an intersubjective connectedness, we value sharing our experiences and inner states. Such moments help us gain small degrees of self-understanding. However, for this to happen our minds (and senses) have to be open. If we are anxious or reluctant, task-minded or defensive, our ability to resonate or to be trusted by the other is limited. Over-reliance on technique or procedure cuts us off from the mental experience of the other. It is only when practitioners create a space in which the client or service user feels potentially safe that these 'present moments' occur. Our mental life, originally fashioned in parent–infant and family–child interaction, continues to be co-created in relationship with others. It is in the matrix of intersubjectivity that we shape the mental experience of others and they shape the inner life of us. This is never a neat, planned process. The co-creation of experience, recognition and understanding is a 'sloppy' business, full of stumblings, reachings-out, steppings-back, gaucheness, false moves, poor turns-of-phrase, and occasional warmth, connection and sudden self-awareness (Stern 2004: 156). Practice is never text-book smooth. And yet in the human desire to be mind-read and to mind-read, however clumsily pursued, lies potential movement and psychological progress.

Psychoanalytic and Psychodynamic Theories and Therapies

One of the basic assumptions of psychodynamic approaches is that early life experiences, particularly with parents, affect emotional development and our mental health, for better or worse.

From the outset, the pioneers in this field believed that talking about thoughts and feelings in the context of a relationship was therapeutic. In the late 19th century, Breuer was treating a young woman, Anna O, who suffered a number of physical symptoms that might have been caused by some previous psychological trauma. During parts of her treatment, including hypnosis, Anna would express strong feelings. Doctor and patient noticed that the symptoms seemed to disappear as Anna gave voice and vent to the emotions. Anna called the treatment her 'talking cure'. She felt 'purged' of her anxieties and as the Greek word for purgation was *katharsis*, so the idea of talking about feelings became known as the 'cathartic method'. Sigmund Freud began to work with Josef Breuer and the beginnings of psychoanalysis – the analysis of the unconscious forces affecting the mind – emerged.

Beneath many mental health problems lie unconscious psychological conflicts. The origins of these conflicts are often to be found in childhood. Treatment requires that these unconscious memories and conflicts be brought back into consciousness. Once back in mind, the traumatic events can be analysed and interpreted in a more conscious and reflective manner by both therapist and patient. In this way, control over the troubling events and the unconscious mental forces can be achieved. The conflict is resolved.

In Freudian terms, psychopathology results from conflicts between the structural parts of the personality: the id, the ego and the superego. The *id* is that part of the mind that is concerned with our basic needs and instinctual drives: food, sex, survival. It pays no attention to reality or social constraint. It operates on the pleasure principle. It gives psychic expression to the body's needs. Needs and desires, when experienced, feel urgent. The id has no sense of right or wrong. It is the reservoir of all our psychic energy, connected as it is with our bodies and our survival.

The *ego* forms as the id comes up against reality. If the id's demands are to be satisfied, the world of other people and things has to be taken into account. The ego operates on the reality principle. If needs are to be met and desires fulfilled, more conscious, reflective and analytical skills have to be employed. The ego therefore acts as the executant of the id, the home of the instinctual drives. In pursuit of its goals, the ego uses thought, calculation and memory. Frustration, in moderation, is therefore essential if the ego is to develop. In this way, the individual learns to delay gratification.

An effective ego helps the individual deal competently with the reality of the environment. People with weak egos have an unrealistic view of the world and feel unable to control their environment. They feel under stress even as they try to negotiate the ups and downs of everyday life. The id, with its infantile demands, is not handled well by those with weak egos. Individuals therefore feel angry, deprived and helpless. When the ego is unable to manage the environment or control the id, the psyche feels overwhelmed and trauma results. Indeed, anything that threatens the ego's integrity is likely to make us feel anxious. In her discussion of psychosocial casework, Hollis believed that social workers should be very mindful of their clients' anxiety states:

> No single factor in treatment is more important than the worker's keeping his finger on the pulse of the client's anxiety . . . What particular things in the client's present or past provoke his anxiousness? How does his anxiety show itself and how does he handle it? In particular: does his anxiety level impel him to unwise acting out? Does it result in increased neurotic or somatic symptomatology? What defenses does he use against it? Is he immobilised? Will he run away from treatment? (Hollis 1964: 315)

The *superego* is the third element of personality structure. As children mature, they are constantly told by parents and other adults what they can and cannot do, what is right and wrong, what is good and bad. The superego is the internalised psychic representation of these moral injunctions, these parental authority figures. These experiences help us develop a conscience. The superego is concerned with social and moral standards. If we have had very severe injunctions about what we can and cannot do, our superegos will play a highly censorious role in not just what we do but also what we think and feel. Feelings of guilt will weigh heavily on our minds.

Our behaviour is the product of the interaction between these three personality structures. When they are in balance, we enjoy good mental health. However, if the ego is weak and feels unable to keep the id's demands in check, anxiety results. If the superego is too dominant, guilt ensues.

The psychodynamic therapist's treatment aim is to: 'uncover the unconscious conflicts that that cause psychological distress, to bring formerly unconscious material into conscious awareness, and to achieve reintegration of the previously repressed material into the total structure of the personality' (Joseph 2001: 72). Successful therapy requires the patient to gain *insight* into the origins and causes of their psychological problems.

A favoured method is to help the patient to talk freely about their thoughts and feelings in a technique known as 'free association'. In the safety of the therapeutic relationship, the patient is encouraged, indeed challenged to explore the repressed conflicts that bubble into consciousness during free association. The therapist seeks to interpret the unconscious mental forces that are causing the psychological conflict and the problem behaviour. Past and present are thereby linked.

Under the challenge and anxiety of treatment, patients show *resistance*. They might try to change the subject or avoid facing up to the therapist's interpretation.

> The aim is not a 'cure' by the expert, but to give patients insight into aspects of themselves and what is going on in their mind, understanding the truth about ourselves is potentially liberating and allows us more control of aspects of our lives. Not surprisingly Freud found that his patients were not keen to know or believe unpleasant things about themselves and improvement was often slowed down by resistance. (Bower 2005: 6)

As we relate with others, we often have thoughts and feelings about them that are actually based on our relationship experiences with someone else, particularly our parents. We therefore feel about or react to them inappropriately. This is the phenomenon of *transference*. Feelings are transferred from a meaningful, typically problematic relationship with someone from the patient's past or present on to the therapist or social care worker. For example, if a patient felt rejected by or anxious to please a parent during childhood, they may unconsciously cast the therapist as rejecting or needy. The therapist will use this insight to help the patient understand the power that unresolved feelings continue to have on present states of mind and current relationships.

Freud attracted many followers, several of whom took his ideas off in new directions, often earning his displeasure. For example, Melanie Klein felt that although the processes of the id were important, children's relationships with their caregivers had a particularly profound effect on psychological development (Klein 1932). The way parents view, feel and think about, understand and interact with their children forms a key, objective part of the child's world and experience. These experiences will help shape the child's mind. This approach became known as the *object-relations* school of thought. In this approach, children 'introject' (incorporate) how others view, think and feel about them. The outside world defines the child's inner world. In this sense, past relationship experiences influence personality formation and the quality of our relationships with others in the present.

Bion developed Klein's idea of projective identification to examine how children learn to handle their own emotions (Bion 1963). The baby's primitive and powerful feeling states are handled, 'contained' and processed by the mother. Over time and with 'good enough' mothering (Winnicott 1965), children internalize their mother's ability to contain and manage their emotions. In this way, children learn to self-regulate their own emotional arousal. Parents who can't or won't contain their children's emotional arousal leave them prey to emotional turmoil. Bower (2005) believes that Bion's model of how mother's help their children achieve emotional regulation provides a useful model for social workers to help them manage their client's emotional states. She suggests that this way of dealing with distress, aggression and fear offers 'a way of understanding how a thoughtful and emotionally receptive stance to clients can have therapeutic value without anything fancy being done' (Bower 2005: 11).

However, even within this perspective, new lines of thinking (and disagreement) opened up, but whether Freud, Klein, Jung, Adler, Erikson, Bion or Bowlby, the common thread is the critical part that childhood experiences are thought to play in personality organization, and how these elements play out in the way we relate with others in the present. If childhood experiences were stressful, painful, frightening or suffocating, there will be a strong chance they will unconsciously disturb and distort the way we feel about and deal with people who are important to us in the present. It is in the context of current relationships that strong feelings and emotional dysregulation are experienced.

Treatments require that these unconscious formative experiences are brought into consciousness where they can be the subject of reflection, analysis and interpretation. The hope is that through the processes of interpretation and insight, feelings of anger or fear, hostility or distress might be recognized and understood before finally being resolved. And critical to the therapeutic process is the relationship with the therapist. It is only if the patient, client or service-user trusts the therapist and feels that the relationship is a safe place to explore raw feeling, that insight and change will take place.

Mentalized Affectivity-Based Treatments

More recently, clinicians who have drawn on psychodynamic theory, developmental attachment theory and the neurosciences have fashioned a range of relationship based emotional supports and treatments. These approaches recognize the importance of 'minds connecting', particularly at the emotional level. Fostering the capacity to *mentalize* is a key part in most treatment and support programmes (Allen and Fonagy 2006: xix). The aim is to help clients and service users 'feel clearly'. Bowlby felt the role of the psychotherapist was to:

> . . . provide the patient with a secure base from which he can explore the various unhappy and painful aspects of his life, past and present, many of which he finds it difficult or perhaps impossible to think about and reconsider without a trusted companion to provide support, encouragement, sympathy, and on occasion, guidance. (Bowlby 1988: 138)

If the emotional brain originally 'hard wired' itself in the context of early close social interactions, then new relationships have the power to nurture and heal the mind (Siegel 2003: 3). Psychotherapy and supportive relationships create environments in which cognition, emotions and behaviour can become integrated at both the neurological, psychological and conscious level. Those who can access and process the full range of their thoughts, feelings and behaviour not only do not need to employ defences, they also have the widest range of options in complex socio-emotional situations. Painful, normally defensively excluded material needs to be accessed, recognized, contained, reflected upon and understood if we are to proceed with skill and sensitivity across the potentially rocky terrain of social relationships.

For example, traumatized service users and patients try to deal with their unbearably painful emotional states by retreat (depression, isolation, dissociation), self-destructive acts (substance abuse, self-harm, suicidal ideation), and destructive acts (aggression, rage). 'Stress', Holmes (2006: 35) reminds us 'is the enemy of mentalization; when anxiety reaches a certain level the mentalizing brain goes offline and moves into survival mode'.

Therapists have to help clients contain and 'stay with' their painful feelings in order to learn how to recognize, contain, process and regulate them. Patients and users are encouraged to use a 'metaphorical pause button by mentalizing; that is we urge them to attend to their emotional state and to sit with their feelings, thereby enriching their sense of self' (Allen 2006: 11). Feeling safe and secure comes from being sensitively understood and emotionally contained. Talking about his work with a male patient who presented with depression and panic attacks associated with post-traumatic memories stemming from sexual assaults in his childhood, Allen describes an example of mentalized-based treatment in practice:

At this juncture [of the treatment], the point of mentalizing became clearer to me: rather than putting the traumatic memories *out* of mind, the patient would be better served by being able to have the memories *in* mind – as emotionally bearable and meaningful experiences, albeit unpleasant and painful. Hence, I suggested that he change strategies: rather than endeavouring to avoid thinking about the traumatic event, he could practice bringing it to mind deliberately without becoming too immersed in it, and then he could use his comforting imagery to relax and put the memory out of mind. He was able to do so and, in the process, developed a sense of control over his mind . . . He no longer feared his own mind . . . (Allen 2006: 4)

In therapy, the therapist holds in her mind the client's mind. The client finds his mind in the mind of the mind-minded, psychologically available therapist. The other then feels 'felt' and understood by the therapist, who seems to have them and their mental state in mind. The individual begins to experience the emotional self more consciously and explicitly.

Individuals who have suffered poor quality care have a limited ability to process and regulate the strong emotions that stressful relationships evoke. Their brains lack complexity. Neurologically and psychologically, they operate in a relatively rigid, compartmentalized way. There is a lack of integration between the way they process cognitive and emotional information. In contrast, emotionally intelligent people have complex brains and very 'open' minds in which the emotional, cognitive, rational, language, memory and somatic parts of the brain communicate and exchange maximum information with each other. This allows the individual to consider a range of options in emotionally demanding situations. Psychotherapy, using an emotionally attuned and responsive relationship, attempts to supply new information and encourage contact between those parts of the brain which have not had a chance to communicate because of previous stresses and traumas. In this way, the cortex begins slowly to become aware of, learn from and regulate the brain's emotional centres.

In the context of the therapeutic meeting or supportive visit, clients and service users feel, say and do things. It is critical that therapists and social workers react in a manner that is contingent, congruent and empathically sensitive. They observe and comment on the user's affective state using reflective dialogue. They track the service user's emotional state as expressed in body language, the voice and the face. Fonagy et al (2002) describe this skill as 'mentalized affectivity': the recognition of one's own and other people's emotional states that affect both parties' feelings, thoughts and behaviour. It is a sophisticated kind of affect regulation. Therapists must foster the client's capacity for 'mentalization', the ability to reflect on one's own and other people emotional states during the to and fro of the relationship. To regulate emotions, clients must first learn to tolerate them. In maintaining an attuned, reflective stance, the therapist:

. . . ultimately enables the client to find himself or herself in the therapist's mind and to integrate this image as part of his or her self-representation. In successful therapy, the client gradually comes to accept that feelings can safely be felt and ideas may be safely thought about. (Fonagy 1998 cited in Allen 2001: 310)

In mentalized affectivity based treatments, the other's emotional, mental and physiological states are recognized, named and mirrored back verbally, facially, in gesture and body posture. The therapist creates a relationship of trust in which the client feels it is safe to explore the mind of the therapist in which the client's own feelings are represented (Bateman and Fonagy 2004: 143).

The technique also believes that the naming of emotions is important. Some people avoid their feelings. They dampen their affects with alcohol or drugs or gambling. Others express feelings that are not congruent with what they are actually feeling. In other cases, emotions easily get out of control. Clients need to gain purchase on their feelings and their possible origin. They also need help to recognize and learn how to handle their arousal. Emotions, when expressed, also need to take account of their impact on others. 'Communicating affects', believe Fonagy et al (2002: 440) 'means that the expression is offered with the expectation of how it will be received by others. One wants the other person(s) not just to know what one feels, but also to understand and perhaps respond to this feeling.'

Recognizing powerful feelings in a safe, containing relationship allows conscious exploration, reflection and the gradual integration of old memories, current triggers and here-and-now thoughts, feelings and behaviours. The sensitively attuned therapist and social care worker allow the client or user to keep in focus and hold in present, short term working memory all those thoughts, emotions and psychological feelings, body sensations, memories, beliefs and behavioural intents just long enough to sense how they might be linked. It is important for service users to try and 'stay with' with their troubling and troublesome feelings, otherwise they stay outside consciousness, beyond understanding and control. Anxious individuals, frightened people, angry clients, depressed patients need emotionally to re-experience causal events without feeling helpless. For example, in the case of trauma, the safe, mind-engaging, containing relationship with the therapist helps the client to realize that 'remembering the trauma is not equivalent to experiencing it again . . . that the experience had a beginning, middle, and an end, and that the event now belongs to one's personal history' (van der Kolk 2003: 189). The final feature of mentalizing is the capacity to remain psychologically open to new experiences, to allow oneself to be influenced by others, to be open to the minds of others in order to think and feel better and more clearly (Allen 2006: 21).

Humanistic Approaches

Although different in many ways, both cognitive behavioural and psychodynamic theories approach the study of human psychology from a scientific, deterministic perspective. In contrast, humanistic-based psychologies value free will, choice and personal responsibility. They believe that we all have the capacity to unlock potential qualities of our being that remain buried beneath the weight of convention, social oppression and denial. So, rather than assess people objectively and seek an explanation, person-centred therapies seek to understand people subjectively. The search for meaning is pursued, not a causal explanation. It is the experience of the other and being in relationship that is the basis of change. The *experiential process* is more important than measuring, classifying and treating particular behaviours and disorders. Nevertheless, in practice, humanistic approaches have many similarities with the broadly defined psychodynamic and mentalization-based treatments.

The ability to show empathy, to see and feel the world from the other's point of view, is a particularly important quality that defines the successful therapist and social worker. However, it is not sufficient just to feel empathic, the understanding reached has to be successfully communicated. To feel understood by another is deeply comforting. To connect with another means that we are not alone, and that maybe it is safe to explore and move on knowing that there is help and support all along the way. The idea that experience can be explored draws its inspiration from the philosopher Husserl's pursuit of knowledge using a phenomenological approach. If we are to understand experience, we must put aside or 'bracket off' all our assumptions, theories, beliefs and expectations. This is what the person-centred counsellor is asking the client to do. 'The act of "bracketing off" or suspending assumptions implies that the phenomenological researcher (or therapist) does not impose his or her theoretical assumptions on experience. As a result, theory in phenomenological approaches to counselling such as the person-centred approach, act more as a general pointer towards potentially significant areas of experience, rather than making any assumptions about the actual content of that experience' (McLeod 1998: 94).

Humanistic psychologies arose in the middle of the 20th century as a 'third force' to match behavioural and psychodynamic psychologies. 'Humanistic therapies,' writes Joseph (2001: 115), 'strive to enable people to accept responsibility for their actions, to become aware of their subjective experiences, and to fulfil their personal potential for personal growth'. The energy for change is to be found within the individual. It is the therapist's task to free that energy. Clients are the experts on their own problems and they are capable of finding their own solution with the support and reflective engagement of the therapist (McLeod 1998: 89).

Perhaps the most familiar of the humanistic therapies is the *person-centred approach*. The defining features of the approach were mapped by Carl Rogers (1942, 1951). Sometimes known as Rogerian therapy, the approach has undergone a number of name changes, including 'non-directive therapy' and 'client-centred therapy', before a consensus settled on 'person-centred' therapy or counselling. Person-centred approaches are relationship-based therapies. And it is in relationships with empathic others that healing takes place.

Humanistic therapies hold a positive view of human beings. There is a strong existential strand running through the approaches: we have no essential nature; we are free to make or 'actualize' who we are if only we can free ourselves of 'bad faith' and embrace freedom and define our selves. Rogers said that at heart we have an *actualizing tendency* in which there is a strong desire to grow, be creative and fulfil our potential. Similarly, Maslow (1968, 1993) saw the pinnacle of human experience as 'self-actualization'. There is also a strong belief that *we all need to be loved and valued by others*. It is the lack of love and feeling de-valued that causes so much personal misery and distress.

People experience problems and distress if, on the one hand they sense that they have more about them then has been realized, and on the other hand, they feel constrained, trapped and bound by other people, their expectations, approval, and qualified acceptance.

People who only feel acknowledged and of value if they act and behave as they believe others wish them to act and behave remain untrue to themselves. Rogers called this 'conditional positive self-regard'. The regard of others is conditional on behaving in a particular way. Parents who belittle their children if they behave too dependently, partners who show great need and distress if they feel uncertain about the other's love, adolescents who are made to feel anxious by their parents if they seek autonomy – all these individuals experience regard but with heavy conditions attached. In this sense, although we are all at the mercy of our social environments, for young children it is the totality of their world that makes them particularly susceptible to experiences of conditional positive regard. If other people are relentlessly critical of us, judge us harshly and generally undermine our independence, our search for positive self-regard becomes ever more agitated and anxious. External judgements and internal experiences feel at odds. What others expect and how we should like to be don't coincide. We feel 'incongruent'. This produces a state of psychological tension which throws our emotions into turmoil. It is feeling incongruent that brings clients to counselling.

> For Rogers, the origins of psychological disturbance lay in the essentially judgemental and invalidating relationships which many people experience not only in their early years but throughout their lives. The healing of such disturbance . . . could best be achieved through the provision of a therapeutic relationship characterized by the elements which were so evidently absent in previous relationships. (Thorne 1997 p 177)

These missing elements need to be experienced in relationship with the therapist or counsellor. If present, the elements, according to the person-centred approach, will be necessary and sufficient to bring about positive change (Truax and Carkhuff 1967). These 'necessary and sufficient conditions', often referred to as the 'core conditions' include:

1. *Unconditional* positive regard (warm involvement with the client).
2. Accurate empathy.
3. Congruence or genuineness.

If these elements are present in good measure, then the client also feels that the relationship is *collaborative* in which a *positive emotional bond* between client and therapist is established. Supported in a relationship of acceptance and trust, the client is encouraged, even challenged to 'stay with' and become more aware of difficult feelings (Rogers 1961). First, feelings are described and then 'owned'. Current feelings are recognized, acknowledged, expressed and explored. With increased understanding, clients can address and regulate their feelings. 'Once this begins to happen the way is open to a radical reordering of the self concept with all that this may entail both for the sense of worth and for behaviour . . . The counsellor's task is not to guide or to direct but patiently to accompany in a way which ensures that clients can breathe a new air which it makes it possible for them to face themselves and their situation without fear' (Thorne 1997: 181). The individual becomes more open to experience and able to evolve, to realize their true self, to *self-actualize,* to live authentically.

Humanistic approaches trust the service user's innate ability to change in their own chosen direction if given the right relationship conditions. From feeling 'how I am now' the user moves towards 'how I would ideally like to be', towards a state of integration and fulfilment. Everyone has the potential to flower if the conditions are right. When we achieve congruence with our selves, the tension melts away and the emotions are re-coloured positive.

Social Support

Although seemingly ordinary and commonplace, the support of family and friends is emotionally very protective. They act as a buffer against the stresses and strains of everyday life. They listen. They can be a shoulder to cry on or a sounding board for plans and ideas. Problems shared are problems halved. Whether we just have one or two close relationships or find ourselves embedded in a wide network of family and friends, we feel connected, we feel we belong. Support, according to Cobb (1976), is when we feel loved and cared for, esteemed and valued, when there is communication and a sense of mutual obligation. At times of need, we feel we can call on others, and they can call on us, emotionally and practically. It is not surprising, therefore, to learn that good social relationships improve our mental health.

One of the key elements of the new positive psychology (the psychology of happiness introduced in Chapter Six) is the presence of satisfying and supportive social relationships. Emotional wellbeing seems to be largely about feeling loved, liked, esteemed, recognized, understood and accepted. Family, friends and feeling socially embedded are key to happiness.

Happiness also includes feeling that we have some control over our lives, that we have a sense of purpose, meaning and can regularly experience what psychologists call 'flow' – the ability to become lost and fully absorbed with what we are doing. A 'state of flow' or happiness occurs when we become lost in the immediacy of experience. 'It is not a matter of waiting for the outside world to bring you pleasures. It's not watching television, or eating chocolate, or winning the lottery. You have to create meaningful activity. This involves a goal, problems to solve, skills that you learn, detailed feedback to evaluate how you are doing' (Oatley 2004 p 148). People in a state of flow become so absorbed in the task at hand they lose all self-consciousness. 'In this sense moments of flow are egoless. Paradoxically, people in flow exhibit a masterly control of what they are doing, their responses perfectly attuned to the changing demands of the task. And although people perform at their peak while in flow, they are unconcerned with how they are doing, with thoughts of success or failure – the sheer pleasure of the act itself is what motivated them' (Goleman 1995: 91). It is when we are in these states of flow that we feel a deep sense of wellbeing and absolute contentment (Csikszentmihalyi 1990).

According to Martin (2005: 50–71) happy people share a number of characteristics of which social connectedness, support, good personal relationships, emotional competence and good communication skills are particularly important. Emotional intelligence improves social competence. Social competence deepens and possibly increases the quality of your personal relationships. Good personal relationships make you feel happy. And happiness improves mental wellbeing and physical health.

In contrast, poor emotional intelligence hampers social relationships. Emotional illiteracy makes it more likely that relationships will be experienced as stressful, conflictual, and difficult. A lack of supportive relationships increases social isolation. Social isolation leads to unhappiness, anxiety and depression. And unhappiness increases the risk of poor mental and physical health.

People's ability to cope with many illnesses and diseases is improved if they enjoy strong and loving social support (Bartlett 1998: 96; Roberts et al 2001: 198). Even simply enjoying personal supports and friendships has been shown to improve your general state of health. Helping families feel less socially isolated, or offering long term home visitation interventions and supports by professionals and individuals from the local community help prevent neglect and maltreatment (Thompson 1995, Olds 2006). Promoting community supports and cohesion allows people to feel socially connected. Older people with little social support have been found to be at higher risk of poor health and even death (Berkman and Syme 1979). If increased emotional support is provided to the most vulnerable members of a community by social care and health workers, mental health, physical health and general wellbeing improve (Cassidy 1999: 71). Older people and other vulnerable groups are less likely to feel alone and more likely to feel safe. Social support which is perceived as available at times of need increases people's feelings of control, that if things go wrong other people are there to help. Feeling in control reduces stress and increases optimism.

Over recent years, social scientists, economists and politicians have recognized that there is something tantalizingly important about happiness, personal relationships and social support. The sum of all these elements they refer to as 'social capital'. Social relationships and a sense of emotional connectedness with others appear to bring great social benefits. Communities that are rich in social capital have lower rates of crime and social unrest. Conversely, they enjoy higher levels of physical health and social cohesion.

Some of the highest rates of happiness, satisfaction and social wellbeing are found in societies in which the economic gap between rich and poor is small (Wilkinson 2000). In countries such as the United States, and increasingly the United Kingdom in which inequality and big differences in income and wealth grow ever greater, social statistics show rising levels of poor mental health, violent crime, dissatisfaction and unhappiness. In grossly unequal societies in which social capital is small, more and more people feel relatively deprived and experience a sense of failure, helplessness and distress.

Conclusion

Running through all of the relationship-oriented treatments and supports is the recognition that human wellbeing is founded on and maintained by good quality relationships. We don't necessarily need an extensive network of family and friends. A few close, meaningful, caring relationships will do. The sadness is that those who cannot regulate their feelings and whose emotional intelligence is poor experience the least satisfactory relationships even though they are the people most in need of people who make them feel valued and understood. It is the job of social workers and social carers, counsellors and therapists to help such people contain and regulate their feelings so that they can stay connected with others. The longer they can remain in 'good enough' relationships with partners, family and friends, and even practitioners themselves, the more they will begin to make emotional sense of themselves. This will reduce feelings of stress. It will increase feelings of being control of their experience. It will raise happiness.

10
The Practitioner Relationship and Emotional Intelligence

Introduction

The psychological self constantly forms and re-forms as we relate with others. From our earliest days as infants to the experience of old age, we recognize and understand ourselves as we engage with parents, family, friends and the community at large. Client, patient and service user views tell us, again and again, that a key ingredient of successful help and effective treatment is the quality of the professional relationship. Practitioners who possess emotional intelligence are most likely to create the most therapeutically positive relationship environments. This final chapter makes the case that emotionally intelligent practitioners are the most socially skilled professionals, likely to relate especially well with service users. Interpersonally skilled and relationship-gifted workers make the most effective and humane practitioners whether the basis of their practice is behavioural, cognitive, task-oriented, psychodynamic or person-centred.

Working with Stress and Under Stress

As we have seen, emotions arise as we unconsciously appraise the world. Emotions give us a quick, fast feel for whether we should proceed, hold back, avoid, or embrace. We feel before we think. Feelings tell us important things about whether we are physically safe, socially accepted, personally connected. It is in relationship with others that we might feel anxious or frightened, angry or sad, jealous or embarrassed, joyous or suspicious. If the emotion is negative, we are likely to employ a variety of psychological defences to protect ourselves from the potential hurt. Anxiety, for example, causes us to become absorbed with our own distress, cutting us off from others.

Despair removes us from the painful effort of mixing with family and friends. Many of our most difficult and intense emotions occur when relationships are not going well.

Working with people who feel under stress is one of social work's basic givens. The bottom line of any social work intervention is the reduction of stress. Relationship problems, poor health, poverty, discrimination, and inadequate housing all cause stress. Practitioners have to address these issues, but the manner and success of that address is coloured by their interpersonal skills. Helping distressed people is itself stressful. Stress and the dysregulating emotions that go with it are therefore endemic to the practice of social work (for example, see Smith 2005 and the need to consider the presence of fear in health and social care work).

If service users are to be helped to recognize and examine their feelings, find the energy to move forward, or regulate their arousal, the strength to achieve these aims is likely to be enhanced if the relationship with the social worker feels safe and containing, accepting and understanding. Social work and social care are essentially relationship-based practices even if many of the explicit techniques and statutory demands impose more formal rules of engagement. Relationships can only be conducted with skill and compassion if the worker is emotionally intelligent.

The Views of Clients and Service Users

What clients, patients and those who use the services of social workers have to say is revealing. Not surprisingly, they review their experiences and their social workers in non-technical language. But what is more interesting, so much of what they have to say casts their experience as an emotional one in which they evaluate the worker and the agency in terms of their personal qualities, empathy and relationship skills (Howe 1993). It is another reminder that people change as they engage with others. They need to trust the worker and feel safe before they can move on and address specific problems, whether those problems are intrapersonal, interpersonal or to do with the business of just trying to live and cope.

The personal qualities of the worker are therefore critical if the service user is to engage with the agency and the help being offered (see for example Drake 1994; Lee and Ayon 2004; Ruch 2005; de

Boer and Coady 2007). If the engagement is successful, the client and worker form a 'therapeutic' or 'helping alliance'. Reviewing their study of parents' views of child and family social workers, Spratt and Callan concluded:

> Irrespective of the nature and source of the referral and the families' previous attitude to social workers, it was their relationship with their particular social worker that parents were to return to again and again . . . in particular their ability to empathise and communication skills. (Spratt and Callan 2004: 217)

Emotionally intelligent social workers help contain service users and their feelings in a relationship that feels safe, safe enough for them to explore. Workers who do not have these skills, or agencies that come across as anxious, defensive or hostile alienate service users. Such agencies and their workers increase distress and anger. They make matters worse. If social workers and their departments are experienced as impersonal, bureaucratic, performance driven, judgemental and punitive, service users will disengage. They might feel abandoned, frightened and angry. Agencies and workers who understand human psychology when it's under stress and practitioners and organizations who are emotionally intelligent not only offer more humane services, they also provide more effective interventions.

If the self formed in the matrix of social relationships, those who experience interpersonal problems seek a return to that matrix in an attempt to find coherence and harmony. However, if relationships are to be restorative then, according to clients, those who provide them must help people feel engaged and secure. It is only then that they can move forward.

The client and consumer literature reveals a number of familiar but nevertheless critical elements that must be present in the social work relationship. They include empathy, containment, acceptance, understanding, and encouragement to explore, make sense and progress. The worker must provide a warm, secure relationship, a 'holding environment', based on mutual respect but one which also expects strenuous effort, and thinking and re-thinking on the part of the client.

In cases in which support and treatment are being offered, social workers should come across as warm and friendly. Service users repeatedly say that they appreciate help that attends to feelings and allows them to think about themselves. The 'warmth factor', as Strupp and colleagues describe it, permeates all client ratings and assessments of what constitutes successful help (Strupp et al 1969: 17). When analysed further, warmth and friendliness appear to be made up of feeling comfortable with the worker, liking and being liked, feeling that the worker is truthful and honest, and that practitioners offering help are emotionally and psychological available. Thinking about their own social work consumer studies, Sainsbury and his colleagues believed that support, encouragement and reliability were overwhelmingly the most helpful aspects of social work involvement over the long term (Sainsbury 1975; Sainsbury et al 1982).

If service users are to explore their feelings they must feel that the professional relationship provides a safe, holding environment. This is facilitated by practitioners who *acknowledge* the user's feelings no matter how distressing or ugly those feelings might be. The feelings are not judged; they are simply *accepted*. This *validates* and *affirms* the feelings. They exist, they have to be faced up to. The feelings are not being denied. Neither user nor social worker are afraid of them even though the feelings may be painful, frightening or highly disturbing.

If the worker can help users contain their feelings and stay with them, the emotions can be thought about, understood and regulated. Mrs Keeling had adopted her son Jason when he was 14 months old. A year later, things were not working out well. She had sought help from a number of agencies before finally becoming a client of a post-adoption support agency:

I began to find looking after Jason more and more difficult. He was an irritable child and I was having problems with him. I visited my doctor about my feelings but he just smiled at me and obviously saw me as a neurotic mother. The adoption agency was not much better and didn't really listen to what I was trying to say. They were too busy trying to reassure me. It was not until I saw the counsellor at the Centre that I could admit, even to myself, that I couldn't seem to love Jason – I didn't even like him. I hated dealing with him physically and I was so upset; I felt so guilty, so distraught. The counsellor gave me time and at last I could say out loud to her – to myself – that I couldn't stand Jason and I felt so, so bad about it but I couldn't make myself feel any different. She just listened and accepted that was just how I was really feeling. There was no point in denying it or giving me silly reassuring noises. It was such a relief to say 'I don't like Jason' and I cried; I couldn't stop crying but it felt better. I could start to face up to what was happening. Pretending was only making things worse. (Howe and Hinings 1989: 21)

To be accepted and recognized bolsters self-esteem. 'I was surprised', said Margaret, a respondent in Woodward's study, 'to find myself able to believe the therapist's positive thoughts about me . . . it had never occurred to me that people would like me . . . I had a poor self-image. Now I think more about and of myself which I know makes me a better person' (Woodward 1988: 86). Social care workers who are not able to tolerate difficult feelings are not helpful.

Once service users feel accepted and understood, safe and contained, they can begin to 'work' on their feelings: their origins; what triggers them; how they affect the self and others; how they can be understood, managed and regulated. This is the beginning of the 'talking' bit of the 'talking cures'. The social worker isn't passive during this stage. She wonders; she might challenge. Service user and worker are in dialogue. A 'conversation' takes place that cements the relationship (Gregson and Holloway 2005). They are trying to make sense of past and present experiences. Service users are trying *to control the meaning of their experience* by ordering and re-structuring their thoughts and feelings, to make better sense of themselves and others.

John, like his parents, was an alcoholic who felt helpless and angry, but with help he began to recognize the cause and effect of his feelings:

. . . as I went through the process I understood how ineffective my mother had been and why she was like that because her childhood was lousy and so I realized that to blame her was not the issue. So the process allowed me to let go of the anger that I experienced about my mother and the damage she did unwittingly. Can't change what happened but I can change me and how I perceive it. (Edmunds 1992: 27)

Service users report 'finding patterns' in their feelings, in their life. Things 'begin to make sense'. A gradual feeling of being in control emerges and with that confidence and self-esteem grow. Control empowers. It overcomes stress. It destroys anxiety. It boosts optimism, the ability to cope and the desire to go forward.

Use of the Self

Implicit in the idea of emotional intelligence is a knowledge of the self, particularly the emotional self. Thus, 'use of the self' is a key aspect of relationship-based practices (for example, see Sudbery 2002). Before the worker can be in touch with the feelings of the client, she must first be able to acknowledge and understand her own emotional states and the power they have to affect her, particularly as she relates with others in need, distress, anger and despair (Shulman 1999: 156). The reference point for an understanding of others is one's self. England (1986) asserts that the 'pervasive use of self is the crucial point of social work' (p 35). And helping, suggests Jordan (1979), is a test of the helper as a person.

The more emotionally aware is the social worker, the more connected she will be with those who use her services and the more open and accurate will be her responses and communications. Nathan, a psychoanalytically-oriented social worker, reflecting on his feelings while dealing with a very stressful mental health referral, provides a sense of how emotional self-awareness can inform good practice.

I went out with doctors and police to do a community Mental Health assessment on a client who had previously been violent. We were confronted by a woman who was screaming at the top of her voice wanting to know why we were there, telling us to get out of her house, etc. I had already begun to look out of the corner of my eye to see just where the police were as I thought she would be violent at any moment. Then I tried to reflect upon what I was experiencing and of course the answer was terror. I wondered if this was how she was feeling. After all, strangers, mostly men, had come into her house and were threatening her very existence. I felt a sense of relief at this insight as I suggested to her that she was terrified by our presence, that she didn't know why we had forced our way into house. I then added that we were worried about her and therefore needed to talk. I suggested sitting down and contin-ued the interview in a much calmer atmosphere even though this ultimately still ended in her being sectioned. (Nathan 1997: 236)

Thus, subjectivity is the touchstone of human experience in which one mind connects and understands another. To know one's self is to know the other and to know the other is to know one's self. Once the connection is made, the self of the service user can form and re-form. The social worker, according to Weigard (cited in England 1986: 46), is like the sculptor who frees the sculpted form from the marble; the worker recognizes the potential of the client and enables him or her to realize that potential.

Although many practitioners will possess high emotional intelli-gence, it can always be developed further. In the stressful world of practice, it needs maintenance and support. Social workers affect and are affected by their clients and their colleagues. The use of self, emotional intelligence and empathy can always be improved during training. Supervision and consultation are essential if practitioners are to remain self-aware and emotionally attuned. Support and supervi-sion for social workers help create a space for 'emotional thinking' (Chamberlayne 2004). Supervision has many elements including containment, case management, information sharing and profes-sional education. However, in its traditional form, supervision contains significant elements of self-reflection and analysis in which social workers think about how clients are affecting them emotionally and how they emotionally affect clients (for example, see Agass 2005).

> . . . the importance of supervision cannot be over-estimated. It would seem essential, not only for the beginner, but also more senior staff. It is important in the first place because it is a way of sharing the heavy responsibility and anxieties aroused in the course of the work; it is a check against distortion due to personal problems; it is a way of counteracting getting in a rut and it provides an opportunity for learning, to develop and further one's insight and skills. (Saltzberger-Wittenberg 1970: 167)

The 'use of self' both as a barometer of events and a therapeutic tool is essential for good practice. Supervision helps keep this key tool sharp and sensitive. If social workers are not to feel angry or fearful, lost or overwhelmed, helpless or despairing, punitive or hostile with cases that are emotionally taxing, there is a great need to reflect on matters with others (Mattinson 1975; Mattinson and Sinclair 1979; Holman et al 2006). Good reflective supervision can help deepen workers' understanding of their own and their service user's psychological condition and mental state so that the therapeutic nature of the relationship between worker and user is maintained.

Organizational cultures that value reflective, emotionally attuned practice also sponsor interventions that are constructive and promote professional mindsets that remain open to case complexity and challenge rather than mindsets that are bureaucratically closed and procedurally driven (Dwyer 2007: 53). It is not only odd but extraordinarily remiss that so few social workers have reflective supervision, particularly given the emotionally demanding and stressful nature of the work. If organizations fail to support, 'hold' and 'contain' their workers, they are in danger of blunting, even destroying the most important resource they have – the emotionally intelligent, available and responsive social worker.

Relationship-Based Social Work

Talking of her own experiences of counselling, France states that 'the quality of the relationship seems to me unquestionably the most valuable part of the experience. It provides the security and motivation indispensable for the more cognitive work in the therapy, and for survival during the really testing moments' (France 1988: 242). Conceiving social work as relationship-based links both emotional intelligence and use of the self. Such approaches are less about what we *do* to service users and more about the relationship we have *with* users.

Relationship-based social work has a distinguished pedigree and goes back a long way in the profession's history. In 1951 Hamilton (pp 27–8) wrote in her book on social casework:

Our most fundamental considerations lie in the concept of human relationships – their importance, their dynamics, their use in treatment ... Relationships can only be experienced directly, although their meaning can be rationally and reflectively assimilated . . . The professional relationship differs from most conventional intercourse largely in the degree to which the aim must be the good of others, in the amount of self-awareness to be attained by the worker, and the techniques to be assimilated and consciously utilised.

In his classic book on the casework relationship, Biestek (1957) identified seven principles on which good practice should be based. They included the purposeful expression of emotion, creating a controlled emotional environment, and being accepting and non-judgemental in one's dealings with the client. Social workers, he felt, should be empathic and be able to use the self in their professional relationship. The casework relationship is 'the dynamic interaction of attitudes and emotions between the caseworker and the client, with the purpose of helping the client achieve a better adjustment between himself and his environment' (Biestek: 17).

In similar vein, Hollis (1972) believed that social casework was based on the recognition that the interplay of both internal psychological and external factors causes social relationship problems. 'Basic to all casework treatment', she argues, 'is the relationship between worker and client' (Hollis 1972: 228). She recognizes that seeking help and becoming involved with social workers creates feelings of anxiety, even anger which trigger a range of defensive behaviours. Service users who have had unhappy relationship histories with parents, partners and professionals will bring these negative experiences and expectations to the new encounter. One of the major skills of a social worker is to recognize and understand these relationship dynamics. Meeting users with acceptance and understanding, empathy and kindness, attunement and containment disconfirms the service user's expectations. The feelings and behaviours that are generated in the worker–client relationship become material that can be used by the worker to help the client explore and understand their psychological and emotional selves as they deal with their environment and other people. If all goes well, such a relationship will gradually lead to a lowering of defences and a growing openness to reflect and change (Lee and Ayon 2004; Ruch 2005).

The relationship flame has been kept burning bright by a steady number of key social welfare thinkers, many working in a Kleinian, object-relations tradition (for example, Cooper and Lousada 2005; Dwyer 2007; Froggett 2002; Hoggett, 2000). The *Journal of Social Work Practice* offers a valuable outlet for much current relationship-based thinking (for example, Hingley-Jones and Mandin 2007; Mandin 2007. A recent attempt to recognize the importance of the social work relationship has been developed by Trevithick (2003). She spells out the importance of relationship-based social work in eight areas of practice including creating a facilitative environment, assessment, support, holding and containing anxieties in times of stress and crises, and providing a foundation for capacity building (Trevithick 2003: 167). She highlights the misery, pain, despair and emptiness that many people suffer when they experience relationship difficulties. The social worker can help provide a relationship in which these feelings can be addressed. The provision of a 'corrective emotional experience' helps 're-energize' the client. Similar ideas are expressed by Sudbery (2002). He gives a nice example of the importance of the social work relationship for Mandy who was anxious that the service she was receiving would be withdrawn:

> Although she had experienced grave practical problems in her life, and had made use of many material services, the reason she gave why she needed her worker was that 'she talks to me, helps me out with my problems – she helps me when I'm feeling down and upset – she helps me be good with my baby'. This (relationship-based) service was needed because in the words of the letter 'If I didn't have nobody I just lose my rag. I lost my children cause I lost my rag. I've got another one, I'm keeping and I'm happy.' (Sudbery 2002: 151)

Grenier (2006) provides a moving study of the emotional needs and experiences of 'frail' older women for whom feelings of loss, grief, anxiety, regret, anger, sadness and fear are real and immediate as their bodies decline and death is suddenly on the near horizon. In the words of Dylan Thomas, they continue to 'rage, rage against the dying light' (Thomas 1937/1971). Companionship and intimacy remain powerful human needs throughout the life course. Grenier makes a compelling case for the value of therapeutic and relationship-based care work with this service user group. She talks about Alice and her growing frailty.

[Alice] talks candidly about her restricted living space – her laundry is now in the kitchen and boxes of diapers clutter her space. Walk rails and adaptive equipment are installed in the home and bathroom. She talks about her body and the way she finds it difficult to do the things that she did before. Her body is a source of embarrassment and shame at times – especially her incontinence. 'My body didn't use to do this', she says. She also talks about the emotional process of adapting: 'I can't adapt – I don't know who I am anymore'. (Grenier 2006: 302)

Grenier points out that the services provided tend to be instrumental, practical and functional, focusing on care and safety, which are needed but fail to connect with Alice's troubled feelings about what is happening to her and her body. She argues that practice has to 'reincorporate emotional experiences and meaning into care encounters', that there is need for social care work to recover its therapeutic roots (Grenier 2006: 306; also see Evans and Garner 2004). Meeting older people's emotional needs, she insists, helps reduce their anxiety and adds immeasurably to the quality of their life.

Emotionally Intelligent Organizations

Relationship skills, argues Morrison (2007) in his paper on the part that emotional intelligence should play in social work, are 'equally important for supervisors, administrators, leaders and managers' (p 249). Emotionally intelligent managers and team leaders induce more co-operation, harmony and creativity in their front-line practitioners. People think more laterally. Teams behave in a more inclusive, flexible, innovative and less hide-bound way. And even though their practices may appear less efficient in terms of time spent on problems and cases, service user satisfaction tends to be higher. When working with people and their needs, effective work is rarely quick work (Salovey et al 2004).

Teams, departments and organizations develop their own emotional climate that can affect mood and morale for good or ill (Goleman et al 2002). Emotionally intelligent management has to recognize that key personnel can affect the emotional tone of everyone else. It is therefore critical to avoid the spread of negative emotions such as anger, aggression, cynicism, anxiety and defensiveness if social work and social care are to be practised with compassion and emotional intelligence.

Anxious managers, aggressive leaders, and defensive supervisors sap optimism and positivity. An unhappy workforce is not only less productive it is less effective. In social care work, anxious practitioners and stressed employees increase service user dissatisfaction leading to poorer outcomes and, perversely, increased referral rates.

Equally contagious are social workers and managers who are emotionally positive and optimistic. They create climates of goodwill, generosity and co-operation (Morrison 2007: 257–8 citing the work of Goleman et al 2002 and Isen 2000). Organizations benefit from the increased productivity, satisfaction, teamwork, and organizational commitment of emotionally intelligent persons. When managers pay more attention to employees and show more concern for their wellbeing, both satisfaction and performance increase.

In the human services, strong arguments are made that if good quality practice requires emotionally intelligent workers, then workers should be selected and appointed on the basis of their emotional intelligence. To a modest degree, emotional intelligence can be improved through training but it has to be acknowledged that in any given population there is a natural distribution of talent, with some people being stronger on what Baron-Cohen (2004) calls systematizing skills associated with jobs such as engineering and information technology and empathizing skills found in nursing, social work, medicine and counselling. Significant numbers of people possess both types of skill in equal measure, but many others are predominantly either 'systematizers' or emotionally intelligent 'empathizers'.

However, Clarke (2006) believes that emotional intelligence can be enhanced, not so much by formal training programmes, but more through workplace analysis and reflection. Observing hospice workers, he noticed that emotional intelligence grew over time as practitioners discussed with colleagues the complex, demanding emotional issues that were part and parcel of their day-to-day work. On the job, experiential learning seems to be much more effective in helping workers improve their emotional intelligence (eg Freshwater and Stickley 2004; Moriarty and Buckley 2003). Good quality supervision, mentoring and skilled management are also key if workplace learning is to be successful. In many occupations, particularly those in social and health care, emotional intelligence seems to improve the quality of the professional relationship, problem-solving, decision-making and clinical practice (Akerjordet and Severinsson 2004; Clarke and Wilcoxson, 2001; David et al 2003).

The Crooked Timber of Humanity

The philosopher Immanuel Kant wrote that 'Out of the crooked timber of humanity no straight thing was ever made.' Isaiah Berlin, quoting Kant, used this insight to examine why men of reason so often end up doing harm to others. The dogged pursuit of rational thought that ignores men's and women's complex natures and elaborate emotional make-up can lead to authoritarian practices. 'To force people into the neat uniforms demanded by dogmatically believed-in schemes is almost always the road to inhumanity. We can only do what we can: but that we must do, against difficulties' (Berlin 1991: 19).

Those who believe that reason has given them the answer to how we should live and relate, and who then set about imposing their reasoned answer on all who come under their power, these people bend minds and force lives to their way of thinking. Berlin believes that such people and their regimes always end up being totalitarian. With deep irony, ideals decay into ideology, rational thought finds itself attacking individuality and difference, reason becomes intolerant of feeling and sentiment. Rational bureaucracies and scientific management run the risk of destroying the true engine of change and effective practice – the emotionally intelligent social worker.

Perhaps more worrying still, many organizations recognize the importance of the 'emotional appearance' of front-line workers for customer manipulation or satisfaction. Flight attendants, supermarket check-out personnel, waiters and waitresses have to act in a friendly, helpful manner even when they feel anything but friendly or helpful. Discrepancies between what is emotionally shown on the outside and felt on the inside can cause stress. Emotions are defined as one of the products or services delivered by the organization. Hochschild (1983) called this the commercialization or 'commodification' of human feeling by large corporations in which emotion is sold as 'labour' – *emotional labour*. The emotions need not be sincere or genuine but they must be expressed, and having been expressed, the emotional performance can be measured and assessed for its impact. The workforce's emotions become prescribed, managed and monitored. Goffman (1959) called this 'impression management'.

Mood regulation and control lie behind these practices. A number of observers of health and social care have witnessed the introduction of 'emotional labour' into the required practice of nurses, social workers and other welfare practitioners. A nice case example is offered by Gorman in her critical examination of the skill needs of care managers as they work with service users. Ironically, in this process, the social work relationship is lost and this is a matter of regret for many care managers:

> I don't have time to sit and talk with the person I am assessing for services. Care management has altered professional identity so that the therapeutic element and the skills one considered to be integral to (social work) practice barely apply. Brokerage, accountancy and political manoeuvring are far more relevant. (Gorman 2000: 154)

Working with people demands an understanding that we are the products of our own unique relationship history and the long, complex emotional journeys that define those histories. The developmental pathways that we each follow are never straight and the many twists and turns in our relationship fortunes create the crooked timber out of which emotionally we are made. The tendency to want to tidy up and legislate away the messiness of human behaviour and social relationships is present throughout the human and social care services. In the eyes of reason we are all irremediably flawed, worker and user alike. To iron out and control the inherent unpredictability that occurs when emotional beings meet and relate, particularly when they are under stress, the men and women of reason, the politicians and policy makers, the managers and inspectors seek to straight-jacket unconformity and resistance by laying down laws, regulating behaviour, producing guidelines, setting up targets and measuring performance. But we can devise no system of rational practice that will entirely succeed, on grounds of simple humanity, by ignoring the crooked timber of our nature. This de-humanization of the people-based services alienates and angers users and increases the stress and anxiety of front-line workers. The emotional temperature rises and the skills to handle the heat decrease.

These are not new thoughts. The critiques and anxieties have been around for a long while but largely ignored. Here are King and Trowell – a lawyer and a psychotherapist – in 1992 despairing of the increasing use of law and statute to deal with child and family distress rather than the skills of the caseworker:

> What we have experienced in recent years is the emergence of law as the dominant institution for the ordering of any intervention in relations between parents, and the extension, through Rules, Regulations and Guidelines, of legal concepts and procedures to cover every aspect of child welfare and protection . . . it is necessary for the law to maintain the myth of rationality even if it conflicts with people's actual experience of the way that families, social services departments, the police and the courts operate in practice, but the maintenance of the myth is not necessarily beneficial to children's interests. (King and Trowell 1992: 128)

They observe that although the legal system is based on notions of social justice and reasonable behaviour, it can nevertheless lead to injustices and a lack of humanity. Rational practices suppress the emotional reality of people trying to cope under stress. The courtroom replaces the clinic. Psychological complexity loses out to procedural correctness. But bureaucratic responses tend to make matters worse in matters of passion. And when matters get worse, when clients get angry, disengage and disappear, despair and destroy, bureaucracies can only respond by meting out more of the same – more plans, more agreements, more threats, more brief and task-focused interventions with no heed paid to the psychological past or the emotional present.

Of course, people, particularly when stress levels are low, can think reflectively and behave rationally. But under increasing stress, anxiety increases. Emotionally intelligent practice prefers to *understand* what is happening to people rather than discipline them into responsibility and good behaviour. When working with people it is better to *make sense* than to *impose* order. Interpretation is better than legislation (Bauman 1987). While reason demands logic and detachment, the human spirit thrives on involvement, relationships and a determination to embrace the tangle of experience (Howe and Hinings 1995). Just as carpenters have to work with the grain of crooked timbers, so social workers must deal skilfully with the weft and warp of human emotion. To ignore this most defining feature of our human make-up is to do harm.

Conclusion

Relationships are complex. It is not surprising therefore to discover that any practice in this field is bound to be difficult, thought provoking, affect-laden and intellectually demanding. It can hardly be left to the rigidities of 'documents, devices and drilled people' (Law 1986). If we are to recover compassion, we need not only emotionally intelligent social workers but also emotionally intelligent organizations which must include those who manage and legislate for them. We need to see people in the context of their relationships and not as discrete, essentially isolated, entirely rational agents so beloved of libertarian thinkers. Emotionally intelligent people are more likely to be happy, and happy people are more likely to approach work positively showing creativity, greater productivity and commitment.

If we can be intelligent *about* emotions – what they are, why we have them, how they affect us – we can be more intelligent *with* them. Social work practises in a world in which emotions run high, out-of-control, or off-track. The emotionally intelligent social worker recognizes the emotional nature of her work and the emotional impact that it has on the self and others. It is in the intelligent use of emotions and understanding the part that emotions play in all our lives, that effective practice and psychological wellbeing occur. Affect regulation lies at the heart of all successful treatments, supports and interventions. This being the case, the regulation of affect is the core skill of the emotionally intelligent social worker.

Bibliography

Adolphs, R. and Damasio A. R. (2001) The interaction of affect and cognition: a neurobiological perspective. In J. P. Forgas (Ed.) *Handbook of Affect and Social Cognition.* New Jersey: Lawrence Erlbaum Associates, pp 27–49.

Agass, D. (2005) The containing function of supervision in working with abuse. In M. Bower (Ed.) *Psychoanalytic Theory for Social Work Practice: Thinking Under Fire.* London: Routledge, pp 185–96.

Akerjordet, K. and Severinsson, E. (2004) Emotional intelligence in mental health nursing talking about practice. *International Journal of Mental Health Nursing* 13, pp 164–70.

Allen, J. (2001) *Traumatic Relationships and Serious Mental Disorders.* Chichester: Wiley.

Allen, J. (2006) Mentalizing in practice. In J. Allen and P. Fonagy (Eds.) *Handbook of Mentalization-Based Treatment.* Chichester: Wiley, pp 3–30.

Allen, J. and Fonagy, P. (2006) *Preface.* In J. Allen and P. Fonagy (Eds.) *Handbook of Mentalization-Based Treatment.* Chichester: Wiley, pp xv–xxi.

Almada, S. J., Zonderman, A. B., Shekelle, R. B. and Dyer, A. R. (1991) Neuroticism and cynicism and risk of death in middle-aged men: The Western Electric Study. *Psychosomatic Medicine.* 53, pp 165–75.

Argyle, M. (2001) *The Psychology of Happiness.* 2nd ed. London: Routledge.

Balbernie, R. (2001) Circuits and circumstances: the early neurobiological consequences of early relationship experiences and how they shape later behaviour. *Journal of Child Psychotherapy* 27(3), pp 237–55.

Bandura, A. (1997) *Self-Efficacy: The Exercise of Control.* New York: W. H. Freeman and Company.

Baron-Cohen, S. (1995) *Mindblindness: An Essay on Autism and Theory of Mind.* Cambridge, MA: MIT Press. In J. Allen and P. Fonagy (Eds.) *Handbook of Mentalization-Based Treatment.* Chichester: Wiley, pp 3–30.

Baron-Cohen, S. (2004) *The Essential Difference.* London: Penguin.

Baron-Cohen, S., Wheelwright, S. and Hill, J. (2001) The 'Reading of the mind in the eyes' test, revised version: a study with normal adults and adults with Asperger Syndrome or high functioning autism. *Journal of Child Psychology and Psychology*, 42, pp 241–52.

Bartlett, D. (1998) *Stress: Perspectives and Processes.* Buckingham: Open University Press.

Bateman, A., and Fonagy, P. (2004) *Psychotherapy for Borderline Personality Disorder.* Oxford: Oxford University Press.

Bauman, Z. (1987) *Legislators and Interpreters: On Modernity, Post-Modernity and Intellectuals.* Oxford: Polity Press.

Beck, A. T., Rush, A. J., Shaw, B. F. and Emery, G. (1979) *Cognitive Therapy of Depression.* New York: Guilford Press.

Beck, A. T. and Emery, G. (1985) *Anxiety Disorders and Phobias: A Cognitive Perspective.* New York: Basic Books.

Beck, A. T. and Weishaar, M. (1989) Cognitive therapy. In Freeman, A., Simon, K. M., Beutler, L. E. and Arkowitz, H. (Eds.) *Comprehensive Handbook of Cognitive Therapy.* New York: Plenum Press, pp 469–98.

Beeghly, M. and Cicchetti, D. (1994) Child maltreatment, attachment and the self system: emergence of an internal state lexicon in toddlers at high social risk. *Developmental Psychopathology*, 6, pp 5–30.

Berkman, L. F. and Syme, S. L. (1979) Social networks, host resistances, and mortality: a nine-year follow-up study of Alameda County residents. *American Journal of Epidemiology*, 109, pp 186–204.

Berlin, I. (1991) *The Crooked Timber of Humanity.* London: Fontana.

Biestek, F. P. (1957) *The Casework Relationship.* London: Allen and Unwin.

Bion, W. R. (1963) *Elements of Psycho-Analysis,* London: Heinemann.

Bjorklund, D. E. and Harnishfeger, K. K. (1995) The evolution of inhibition mechanisms and their role in human cognition and behavior. In F. N. Dempster and C. J. Brainerd (Eds.) *Interference and Inhibition in Cognition.* San Diego: Academic Press, pp 141–73.

Blackburn, I. D. M. and Davidson, K. (1995) *Cognitive Therapy for Depression and Anxiety* Oxford: Blackwell Science.

Bower, M. (2005) Psychoanalytic theories for social work practice. In M. Bower (Ed). *Psychoanalytic Theory for Social Work Practice: Thinking Under Fire.* London: Routledge, pp 3–14.

Bowlby, J. (1969) *Attachment and Loss: Volume 1: Attachment.* Hogarth Press, London.

Bowlby, J. (1979) *The Making and Breaking of Affectional Bonds.* London: Tavistock.

Bowlby, J. (1980) *Attachment and Loss: Volume 3: Loss.* London: Hogarth Press.

Bowlby, J. (1988) *A Secure Base: Parent–Child Attachment and Healthy Human Development.* New York: Basic Books.

Brazeleton, T. B. (1992) *Head Start: The Emotional Foundations of School Readiness.* Arlington, VA: National Center for Clinical Infant Programs.

Brown, G. (1998) Loss and depressive disorders. In B. P. Dohrenwend (Ed.) *Adversity, Stress, and Psychopathology.* San Diego, CA: Academic Press, pp 358–70.

Brown, G. and Harris, T. (1978) *Social Origins of Depression: A Study of Psychiatric Disorder in Women.* London: Tavistock.

Brown, G., Monck, E., Carstairs, G. and Wing, J. (1962) Influence of family life on the course of schizophrenic illness. *British Journal of Preventative Medicine*, 16, pp 55–68.

Brown, J. R. and Dunn, J. (1996) Continuities in emotion understanding from 3–6 yrs. *Child Development*, 67, pp 789–802.

Buckner, J. C., Mezzacappa, E. and Beardslee, W. R. (2003) Characteristics of resilient youths living in poverty: The role of self-regulatory processes. *Development and Psychopathology*, 15, pp 139–62.

Burnett, R. and Roberts. R. (Eds.) (2004) *What Works in Probation and Youth Justice: Developing Evidence-Based Practice*. Cullompton: Willan Publishing.

Caspi, A., Elder, G. H. and Bem, D. J. (1987) Moving against the world: life course patterns of explosive children. *Developmental Psychology*, 23, pp 308–13.

Caspi, A., Elder, G. H. and Bem, D. J. (1988) Moving away from the world: life course patterns of shy children. *Developmental Psychology*, 24, pp 824–31.

Caspi, A., McClay, J., Mofitt, T. E, Mill, J., Martin, J., Craig, I. W., Taylor, A. and Poulton, R. (2002) Role of genotype in the cycle of violence in maltreated children. *Science*, 297, pp 851–4.

Caspi, A., Sugden, K., Moffitt, T. E., Taylor, A., Craig, I. W., Harrington, H., McClay, J., Mill, J., Martin, J., Braithwaite, A. and Poulton, R. (2003) Influence on life stress on depression: moderation by a polymorphism in the 5-HTT gene. *Science*, 301, pp 386–9.

Cassidy, T. (1999) *Stress, Cognition and Health*. London: Routledge.

Chamberlayne, P. (2004) Emotional retreat and social exclusion: towards biographical methods in professional training. *Journal of Social Work Practice*, 18(3), pp 337–50.

Clarke, C. and Wilcoxson, J. (2001) Professional and organisational learning: analysing the relationship with the development of practice. *Journal of Advanced Nursing*, 34(2), pp 264–72.

Clarke, N. (2006) Developing emotional intelligence through workplace learning: findings from a case study in healthcare. *Human Resources Development International*, 9(4), pp 447–65.

Cobb, S. (1976) Social support as a moderator of life stress. *Psychosomatic Medicine* 38, pp 300–13.

Cohen, S., Doyle, W. J., Skoner, D. P., Rabin, B. S. and Gwaltney, J. M. (1997) Social ties and susceptibility to the common cold. *Journal American Medical Association*, 277(24), pp 1940–4.

Cohen, S., Kaplan, J. R. and Cunnick, J. E. (1992) Chronic social stress, affiliation and cellular immune response in nonhuman primates, *Psychological Science* 3, pp 301–4.

Cohen, S., Tyrell, D. A., and Smith, A. P. (1991) Psychological stress and susceptibility to the common cold. *New England Journal of Medicine*, 325, pp 606–12.

Collingwood, R. G. (1938) *The Principles of Art.* Oxford: Oxford University Press.

Cooper, A. and Lousada, J. (2005) *Borderline Welfare: Feeling and Fear of Feeling in Modern Welfare.* London: Karnac.

Cozolino, L. (2006) *The Neuroscience of Human Relationships: Attachment and the Development of the Social Brain.* New York: W. W. Norton.

Crozier, R. (2006) *Blushing and the Social Emotions: The Self Unmasked.* Basingstoke: Palgrave Macmillan.

Csikszentmihalyi, M. (1990) *Flow: The Psychology of Optimal Experience.* New York: HarperCollins.

Csikszentmihalyi, M. (1998) *Living Well: The Psychology of Everyday Life.* London: Phoenix.

Damasio, A. (1999) *The Feeling of What Happens: Body and Emotion in the Making of Consciousness.* New York: Harcourt.

Danner, D. D. and Snowdon, D. A. (2001) Positive emotions in early life and longevity: findings from the nun study. *Journal of Personality and Social Psychology,* 80(5), pp 804–13.

Darwin, C. (1872/1965) *The Expression of the Emotions in Man and Animals.* Chicago, University of Chicago Press.

David, D. Evans, M., and Jadad, A. (2003) The case for knowledge translation: shortening the journey from evidence to effect. *British Medical Journal,* 327, pp 33–5.

De Bellis, M. (2001) Developmental traumatology: the psychobiological development of maltreated children and its implications for research, treatment, and policy. *Development and Psychopathology,* 13: 539–64.

de Boer, C. and Coady, N. (2007) Good helping relationships in child welfare: learning from stories of success. *Child and Family Social Work,* 12(1), pp 32–42.

Denham, S. A., McKinley, M., Couchoud, E. A. and Holt, R. (1990). Emotional and behavioral predictors of preschool peer ratings. *Child Development,* 61, pp 1145–52.

Dennett, D. (1987) *The Intentional Stance.* Cambridge, Mass.: MIT Press.

Drake, B. (1994) Relationship competencies in child welfare services. *Social Work,* 39, pp 595–602.

Dunbar, R. I. M. (1993). Coevolution of neocortical size, group size, and language in humans. *Behavioral and Brain Sciences,* 16, pp 681–735.

Dunn, J., Brown, J. and Beardsall, L. (1991) Family talk about feeling states and children's later understanding of others' emotions. *Developmental Psychology,* 27(3), pp 448–55.

Dwyer, S. (2007) The emotional impact of social work practice. *Journal of Social Work Practice,* 21(1), pp 49–60.

Edmunds, M. (1992) *Co-dependency and Counselling.* Unpublished MSW interview transcripts, University of East Anglia, Norwich.

Eibl-Eibesfeldt, I. (1973) The expressive behaviour of the deaf-and-blind born. In M. von Cranach and I. Vine (Eds.) *Social Communication and Movement*. New York: Academic Press, pp 163–94.

Ekman, P. (1989) The argument and the evidence about universals in facial expressions of emotion. In H. Wagner and A. Manstead (Eds.) *Handbook of Social Psychophysiology*. Chichester: Wiley, pp 143–64.

Ekman, P. (1992) An argument for basic emotions. *Cognition and Emotion*, 6, pp 169–200.

Ellis, A. (1962) *Reason and Emotion in Psychotherapy*. New York: Stuart.

England, H. (1986) *Social Work as Art: Making Sense for Good Practice*. London: Allen and Unwin.

Evans, D. (2001) *Emotion: The Science of Sentiment*. Oxford: Oxford University Press.

Evans, D. and Cruse, P. (2004) Introduction. In D. Evans and P. Cruse (Eds.) *Emotion, Evolution, and Rationality*. Oxford: Oxford University Press, pp xi–xviii.

Evans, S. and Garner, J. (2004) *Talking Over the Years: A Handbook of Dynamic Therapy with Older Adults*. New York: Brunner-Routledge.

Eyberg, S. M., Boggs, S. R. and Pelham, W. (1995) Parent–child interaction therapy: A psychosocial model for the treatment of young children with conduct problem behaviour and their families, *Psychological Bulletin* 31, pp 83–91.

Fahlberg, V. (1991) *The Child's Journey Through Placement*. Indianapolis: Perspectives Press.

Feldman Barrett, L. and Gross, J. J. (2001) Emotional intelligence: a process model of emotion representation and regulation. In T. J. Mayne and G. A. Bonanno (Eds.), *Emotions: Current Issues and Future Directions*. New York: Guilford Press, pp 286–310.

Field, T., Woodson, R., Greenberg, R. and Cohen, D. (1982). Discrimination and behavior in neonates. *Science*, 218, pp 179–81.

Fischer, A. H., Manstead, A., Evers, C., Timmers, M. and Valk, G. (2004) Motives and norms underlying emotion regulation. In P. Philippott and R. S. Feldman (Eds.) *The Regulation of Emotion*. Mahweh, NJ: Lawrence Erlbaum Associates, pp 187–210.

Fine, S. E., Izard, C. E., Mostow, A. J., Trentacosta, C. J. and Ackerman, B. P. (2003) First grade emotion knowledge as a predictor of fifth grade self-reported internalizing behaviours in children from economically disadvantaged families. *Development and Psychopathology*, 15, pp 331–42.

Foley, D. L., Eaves, L. J., Wormley, B., Silberg, J. L., Maes, H. H., Kuhn, J., et al (2004) Childhood adversity, monoamine oxidase A genotype and conduct disorder. *Archives of General Psychiatry* 61, pp 738–44.

Fonagy, P. (2000) Attachment in infancy and the problem of conduct disorders in adolescence: the role of reflective function. Plenary address to the

International Association of Adolescent Psychiatry, San Francisco, January.

Fonagy, P. (2001) Foreword. In J. Allen *Traumatic Relationships and Serious Mental Disorders*. Chichester: John Wiley, pp xv–xvii.

Fonagy, P., Gergely, G., Jurist, E. and Target, M. (2002) *Affect Regulation, Mentalization and the Development of the Self*. New York: Other Press.

Forehand, R. and McMahon, R. J. (1981) *Helping the Noncompliant Child: A Clinician's Guide to Parent Training*. New York: Guilford Press.

Forgas, J. P. (2001a) Preface. In J. P. Forgas (Ed.) *Handbook of Affect and Social Cognition*. New Jersey: Lawrence Erlbaum Associates, pp xv–xviii.

Forgas, J. P. (2001b) Affect, cognition, and interpersonal behaviour: the mediating role of processing strategies. In J. P. Forgas (Ed.) *Handbook of Affect and Social Cognition*. New Jersey: Lawrence Erlbaum Associates, pp 293–318.

Forster, M. (2007) *Keeping the World Away*. London: Vintage Books.

France, A. (1988) *Consuming Psychotherapy*. Free Association Books: London.

Freshwater, D. and Stickley, T. (2004) The heart of the art: emotional intelligence in nurse education. *Nursing Enquiry*, 11(2), pp 91–8.

Freud, S. (1915) Mourning and melancholia. *The Standard Edition of the Complete Psychological Works of Sigmund Freud*. London: Hogarth Press, 14, pp 239–90.

Frijda, N. H. (1986) *The Emotions*. Cambridge University Press: Cambridge.

Frith, U. (1991) *Autism and Asperger's Syndrome*. Cambridge: Cambridge University Press.

Froggett, L. (2002) *Love, Hate and Welfare: Psychosocial Approaches to Policy and Practice*. Policy Press: Bristol.

Gardner, H. (1983) *Frames of Mind: The Theory of Multiple Intelligences*. New York: Basic Books.

Gardner, H. (1993) *Multiple Intelligences: The Theory in Practice*. New York: Basic Books.

Gerhardt, S. (2004) *Why Love Matters: How Affection Shapes a Baby's Brain* London: Brunner-Routledge.

Goffman, E. (1959) *The Presentation of Self in Everyday Life*. New York: Doubleday and Co.

Goleman, D. (1995) *Emotional Intelligence*. New York: Bantum Books.

Goleman, D., Boyatis, R. and McKee, A. (2002) *Primal Leadership*. Boston: Harvard University Press.

Gorenstein, E. E. and Comer, R. J. (2002) *Case Studies in Abnormal Psychology*. New York: Worth Publishers.

Gorman, H. (2000) Winning hearts and minds? Emotional labour and learning for care management. *Journal of Social Work Practice*, 14(2), pp 149–58.

Gottman, J. M. and Levenson, R. W. (1992) Marital processes predictive of later dissolution: behaviour, psychology and health. *Journal of Personality and Social Psychology*, 63, pp 221–33.

Greenfield, S. (1998) *The Human Brain*. Phoenix, London.

Gregson, M. and Holloway, M. (2005) Language and the shaping of social work. *British Journal of Social Work*, 35(1), pp 37–53.

Grenier, A. (2006) The distinction between being and feeling frail: exploring emotional experiences in health and social care. *Journal of Social Work Practice*, 20(3), pp 299–313.

Hamilton, G. (1951) *The Theory and Practice of Social Case Work* (2nd ed.). New York: Columbia University Press.

Hampton, S. (2004) Adaptations for nothing in particular. *Journal for the Theory of Social Behaviour*, pp 35–53.

Hankin, B. L., Abela, J. R. Z., Auerbah, R. P., McWhinnie, C. M. and Skitch, S. A. (2005) Development of behavioral problems over the life course. In B. L. Hankin and J. R. Z. Abela (Eds.) *Development of Psychopathology: A Vulnerability-Stress Perspective*. Thousand Oaks: Sage, pp 385–416.

Happé, F. (1996) *Autism*. London: University College London Press.

Harris, J. (1999) Individual differences in understanding emotion: the role of attachment status and psychological discourse. *Attachment and Human Development*, 1(3), pp 325–42.

Haviland, J. and Lelwicka, M. (1987) The induced affect response: 10-week old infants' responses to three emotional expressions. *Developmental Psychology*, 23, pp 97–104.

Hebb, D. O. (1949) *The Organisation of Behavior*. New York: Wiley.

Hein, S. (2006) History and definition of emotional intelligence. http://eqi.org/history/htm 11/01/2006

Hingley-Jones, H. and Mandin, P. (2007) 'Getting to the root of problems': the role of systemic ideas in helping social work students to develop relationship-based practice. *Journal of Social Work Practice*, 21(2), pp 177–91.

Hobson, P. (2002) *The Cradle of Thought: Explorations on the Origin of Thinking*. London: Macmillan.

Hochschild, A. (1983) *The Managed Heart: Commercialisation of Human Feeling*. Berkeley: University of California Press.

Hoggett, P. (2000) *Emotional Life and the Politics of Welfare*. Basingstoke: Macmillan.

Hollis, F. (1972) *Casework: A Psychosocial Therapy* (2nd ed.). New York: Random House.

Holman, C., Meyer, J. and Davenhill, R. (2006) Psychoanalytically informed research in an NHS continuing care unit for older people: exploring and developing staff's work with complex loss and grief. *Journal of Social Work Practice*, 20(3), pp 315–28.

Holmes, J. (2006) Mentalizing from a psychoanalytic perspective: what's new? In J. Allen and P. Fonagy (Eds.) *Handbook of Mentalization-Based Treatment*, Chichester: Wiley, pp 31–49.

Howe, D. (1993) *On Being a Client: Understanding the Process of Counselling and Psychotherapy*. Sage: London.

Howe, D. (2005) *Child Abuse and Neglect: Attachment, Development and Intervention*. Basingstoke: Palgrave Macmillan.

Howe, D. and Hinings, D. (1989) *Adopters and their Families: The Post-Adoption Centre; First Three Years*, Research Report Number 3. Norwich: University of East Anglia.

Howe, D. and Hinings, D. (1995) Reason and emotion in social work practice: managing relationships with difficult clients. *Journal of Social Work Practice*, 9(1), pp 5–14.

Hubel, D. H. and Wiesel, T. N. (1962) Receptive fields, binocular interaction, and functional architecture in the cat's visual cortex. *Journal of Physiology*, 160, pp 106–54.

Hudson, B. and Macdonald, G. (1986) *Behavioural Social Work: An introduction*. London: Macmillan.

Huesman, L. R., Eron, L. D., Lefkowitz, M. and Walder, L. O. (1984) Stability of aggression over time and generations. *Developmental Psychology*, 20, pp 1120–34.

Humphrey, N. (1986) *The Inner Eye*. London: Faber and Faber.

Ironside, V. (2007) *No! I Don't Want to Join a Bookclub*. London: Penguin.

Isen, A. M. (2000) Positive affect and decision making. In M. Lewis and J. Haviland-Jones (Eds.) *The Handbook of Emotions* (2nd ed.). New York: Guilford Press.

Isen, A. M. and Levin, P. F. (1972) The effects of feeling good on helping: cookies and kindness. *Journal of Personality and Social Psychology*, 21, pp 384–8.

Isen, A. M., Rosenzweig, A. S. and Young, M. J. (1991) The influence of positive affect on clinical problem solving. *Medical Decision Making*, 11, pp 221–7.

James. W. (1884/1968) What is an emotion? In M. B. Arnold (Ed.) *The Nature of Emotion*. Harmondsworth: Penguin, pp 17–36.

Jamison, K. R. (1995) *An Unquiet Mind*. London: Picador.

Jenkins, J. M. and Oatley, K. (1996) The development of emotional schemas in children: the processes underlying psychopathology. In W. F. Flack and J. D. Laird (Eds.) *Emotions and Psychopathology*. Oxford: Oxford University Press, pp 45–56.

Jenkins, J. M., Smith, M. A. and Graham, P. (1989) Coping with parental quarrels. *Journal of the American Academy of Child and Adolescent Psychiatry*, 28, pp 182–9.

Johnson, J. G., McGeoch, P. M., Caskey, V. P., Abhary, S. G., Sneed, J. R. and Bornstein, R. F. (2005) The developmental psychopathology of personality disorders. In B. L. Hankin and J. R. Z. Abela (Eds.) *Development of Psychopathology: A Vulnerability-Stress Perspective*. Thousand Oaks: Sage, pp 417–64.

Jordan, B. (1979) *Helping in Social Work*. London: Routledge and Kegan Paul.

Joseph, R. (1999) The neurology of traumatic 'dissociative' amnesia. *Child Abuse and Neglect* , 23(8), pp 715–27.

Joseph, S. (2001) *Psychopathology and Therapeutic Approaches: An Introduction.* Basingstoke: Palgrave Macmillan.

Kagan, J. (1994) *Galen's Prophecy: Temperament in Human Nature.* London: Free Association Books.

Kaufman, J. and Charney, D. (2001) Effects of early stress on brain structure and function: implications for understanding the relationship between child maltreatment and depression. *Development and Psychopathology*, 13, pp 451–71.

Kemper, T. D. (1990) Social relations and emotions: a structural approach. In T. D. Kemper (Ed.) *Research Agendas in the Sociology of Emotions.* Albany, NY: State University of New York University Press, pp 207–37.

Kiecolt-Glaser, J. K., Fisher, L., Ogrocki, P., Stour, J., Speicher, C. and Glaser, R. (1987) Marital quality, maritial disruption, and immune function. *Psychosomatic Medicine*, 49(1), pp 13–34.

Kiecolt-Glaser, J. K., Malarkey, W. B., Chee, M., Newton, T., Cacioppi, J. T., Mao, H. and Glaser, R. (1993) Negative behaviour during marital conflict is associated with immunological down-regulation. *Psychosomatic Medicine*, 55, pp 395–405.

King, M. and Trowell, J. (1992) *Children's Welfare and the Law: The Limits of Legal Intervention*, London: Sage.

Kitayama, S., Karasawa, M. and Mesquita, B. (2004) Collective and personal processes in regulating emotions: emotion and self in Japan and the United States. In P. Philippott and R. S. Feldman (Eds.) *The Regulation of Emotion.* Mahweh, NJ: Lawrence Erlbaum Associates, pp 251–73.

Klein, M. (1932) *The Psychoanalysis of Children*, London: Hogarth.

Kring, A. M. and Werner, K. H. (2004) Emotion regulation and psychopathology. In P. Philippott and R. S. Feldman (Eds.) *The Regulation of Emotion.* Mahweh, NJ: Lawrence Erlbaum Associates, pp 359–85.

Lahey, B. B., McBurnett, K. and Loeber, R. (2000) Are attention-deficit hyper-activity disorder and oppositional defiant disorder developmental precursors to conduct disorder? In A. Sameroff, M. Lewis, and S. Miller (Eds.) *Handbook of Developmental Psychopathology* (2nd ed.). New York: Plenum, pp 431–46.

Law, J. (1986) On the methods of long-distance control: vessels, navigation and the Portugese route to India. In J. Law (Ed.) *Power, Action and Belief: A New Sociology of Knowledge?* London: Routledge, pp 1–25.

Layder, D. (2004) *Emotion in Social Life: The Lost of Heart of Society.* London: Sage.

Lazarus, R. S. and Folkman, S. (1984) *Stress, Appraisal, and Coping.* New York: Springer.

Lee, C. D. and Ayon, C. (2004) Is the client–worker relationship associated with better outcomes in mandated child abuse cases? *Research on Social Work Practice*, 14, pp 351–7.

LeDoux (1998) *The Emotional Brain: The Mysterious Underpinnings of Emotional Life*. London: Weidenfeld and Nicolson.

Lemma, A. (1996) *Introduction to Psychopathology*. Thousand Oaks: Sage.

Lindemann, E. (1944). Symptomatology and management of acute grief. *American Journal of Psychiatry*, 101, pp 141–9.

Loeber, R. and Farrington, D. P. (2000) Young children who commit crime: epidemiology, developmental origins, risk factors, early interventions, and policy implications. *Development and Psychopathology*, 12, pp 737–62.

Lomas, P. (1981) *The Case for a Personal Psychotherapy*. Oxford: Oxford University Press.

Luthar, S. S. (2006) Resilience in development: a synthesis of research across five decades. In D. Cicchetti and D. J. Cohen (Eds.) *Developmental Psychopathology: Volume 3: Risk, Disorder and Adaptation* (2nd ed.). John Wiley and Sons, pp 739–95.

Lutz, C. A. (1988) *Unnatural Emotions: Everyday Sentiments on a Micronesian Atoll and their Challenge to Western Theory*. Chicago: University of Chicago Press.

Lutz, C. A. and White, G. M. (1986) The anthropology of emotions. *Annual Review of Anthropology*, 15, pp 405–36.

MacLean, P. D. (1990) *The Triune Brain in Evolution*. New York: Plenum Press.

Maluccio, A. N. (1979) *Learning from Clients*. Free Press: New York.

Mandin, P. (2007) The contribution of systems and object-relation theories to an understanding of the therapeutic relationship in social work. *Journal of Social Work Practice*, 21(2), pp 149–62.

Martin, P. (2005) *Making People Happy*. London: Harper Perennial.

Martel, Y. (1993) *The Facts Behind the Helsinki Roccamatios*. New York: Harcourt.

Marucha, P. T., Kiecolt-Glaser, J. K. and Favegehi, M. (1998) Mucosal wound healing is impaired by examination stress. *Psychosomatic Medicine*, 60, pp 362–5.

Maslow, A. H. (1968) *Toward a Psychology of Being* (2nd ed.). New York: Harper and Row.

Maslow, A. H. (1993) *The Farther Reaches of Human Nature*. London: Penguin Arkana

Mattinson, J. (1975) *The Reflection Process in Casework Supervision*. London: Institute of Marital Studies.

Mattinson, J. and Sinclair, I. (1979) *Mate and Stalemate*. London: Institute of Marital Studies.

Mayer, J. D. (2001) Emotion, intelligence and emotional intelligence. In J. P. Forgas (Ed.) *Handbook of Affect and Social Cognition*. New Jersey: Lawrence Erlbaum Associates, pp 410–31.

Mayer, J. D. and Salovey, P. (1997) What is emotional intelligence? In P. Salovey and D. Sluyter (Eds.) *Emotional Development and Emotional Intelligence: Implications for Educators.* New York: Basic Books, pp 3–31.

Mayer, J. D., Salovey, P. and Caruso, D. R. (2000) Emotional intelligence as zeitgeist, as personality, and as a mental ability. In R. Bar-On and J. D. A. Parker (Eds.), *The Handbook of Emotional Intelligence.* San Francisco: Jossey Bass, pp 92–117.

Mayer, J. D., Salovey, P. and Caruso, D. R. (2004). Emotional intelligence: theory, findings, and implications. *Psychological Inquiry,* 15(3), pp 197–215.

McLeod, J. (1998) *An Introduction to Counselling* (2nd ed.). Buckingham: Open University Press.

Meins, E. (1997) *Security of Attachment and the Social Development of Cognition.* Hove: Psychology Press.

Meins, E. (1999) Sensitivity, security and internal working models: bridging the transmission gap. *Attachment and Human Development,* 1(3), pp 325–42.

Moffit, T. (1993) Adolescent-limited and life-course persistent antisocial behaviour: a developmental taxonomy. *Psychological Review,* 100, pp 674–701.

Moriarty, P. and Buckley, F. (2003) Increasing team emotional intelligence through process. *Journal of European Industrial Training,* 27(2), pp 2–4.

Morrison, T. (2007). Emotional Intelligence, Emotion and Social Work: Context, Characteristics, Complications and Contribution. *British Journal of Social Work,* 37(2), pp 245–63.

Mowrer, O. (1947) On the dual nature of learning. *Harvard Educational Review* 17, pp 102–48.

Mowrer, O. J. (1960) *Learning Theory and Behavior.* New York: John Wiley and Sons.

Nathan, J. (1997) Psychoanalytic theory. In M. Davies (Ed.) *The Blackwell Companion to Social Work.* Oxford: Blackwell, pp 231–7.

Neubauer, A. and Freudenthaler, H. H. (2005). Models of emotional intelligence. In R. Schulze and R. D. Roberts (Eds.) *Emotional Intelligence: An International Handbook,* Hogrefe, pp 31–50.

Oatley, K. (1998) Emotion. *The Psychologist,* June, pp 285–8.

Oatley, K. (2004). *Emotions: A Brief History.* Oxford: Blackwell.

Oatley, K. and Jenkins, J. M. (1996) *Understanding Emotions.* Oxford: Blackwell.

Oatley, K., Keltner, D. and Jenkins, J. M. (2006) *Understanding Emotions* (2nd ed.). Oxford: Blackwell.

Olds, D. (2006) The nurse–family partnership: an evidence-based preventive intervention. *Infant Mental Health Journal,* 27(1), pp 5–25.

Orlinsky, D. E. and Howard, K. I. (1986) The psychological interior of psychotherapy: explorations with the therapy session reports. In L. Greenberg and W. Pinsof (Eds.) *The Psychotherapeutic Process.* New York: Guilford Press, pp 477–501.

Orlinsky, D. E., Ronnestad, M. H. and Willutski, U. (2004). Fifty years of psychotherapy process-outcome research: continuity and change. In M. J. Lambert (Ed.) *Bergin and Garfield's Handbook of Psychotherapeutic Behavior and Change* (5th ed.). New York: Wiley, pp 307–89.

Parker, J. D. A. (2005) The relevance of emotional intelligence for clinical psychology. In R. Schulze and R. D. Roberts (Eds.) *Emotional Intelligence: An International Handbook*. Hogrefe, pp 271–88.

Parkinson, B. (2004) Unpicking reasonable emotions. In D. Evans and P. Cruse (Eds.) *Emotion, Evolution, and Rationality*. Oxford: Oxford University Press, pp 107–29.

Pascal, B. (1643/1966) *Pensées*. Baltimore: Penguin.

Pavlov, I. (1928) *Lectures on Conditioned Reflexes*. New York: Liveright.

Patterson, G. R. (1976) *Living with Children: New Methods for Parents and Teachers* (revised edition). Champaign, IL: Research Press.

Payne, W. L. (1985) A Study of emotion: developing emotional intelligence. Unpublished doctoral thesis. Cincinnati: The Union Institute, Cincinnati.

Pearlin, L. I. and Schooler, C. (1978) The structure of coping. *Journal of Health and Social Behavior*, 19, pp 2–21.

Perry, B. (1997) Incubated in error: neurodevelopmental factors in the 'cycle of violence'. In J. Osofsky (Ed.) *Children in a Violent Society*, New York: Guilford Press.

Perry, B. D. and Pollard, R. (1998) Homeostasis, stress, trauma, and adaptation: A neurodevelopmental view of childhood trauma. *Child and Adolescent Psychiatric Clinics of North America*, 7(1), pp 33–51.

Pinker, S. (1997) *How the Mind Works*. Harmondsworth: Penguin.

Provine, R. R. (2000) *Laughter: A Scientific Investigation*. New York: Viking Putnam.

Ramachandran, V. (2003) *The Emerging Mind*. London: Profile Books.

Richman, N., Stevenson, J. and Graham, P. J. (1982) *Preschool to School*. London: Academic Press.

Rimé, B., Finkenauer, C., Luminet, O., Zech, E. and Philippot, P. (1998) Social sharing of emotion: new evidence and new questions. *European Review of Social Psychology*, 9, pp 145–89.

Rizzolatti, G., Fadiga, L., Fogassi, L. and Gallese, V. (1999) Resonance behaviours and mirror neurons. *Archives Italiennes de Biologie*, 137, pp 85–100.

Roberts, C. (2004) Offending behaviour programmes: emerging evidence and implications for practice. In R. Burnett and C. Roberts (Eds.) *What Works in Probation and Youth Justice: Developing Evidence-Based Practice*. Cullompton: Willan Publishing, pp 134–58.

Roberts, R., Towell, T. and Golding, J. (2001) *Foundations of Health Psychology*. Basingstoke: Palgrave Macmillan.

Roberts, W. and Strayer, J. (1987) Parent responses to the emotional distress of their children: relations with children's competence. *Developmental Psychology*, 23, pp 415–25.

Robinson, J. (2007) *Deeper than Reason: Emotion and its Role in Literature, Music, and Art.* New York: Clarendon Press.

Rogers, C. R. (1942) *Counseling and Psychotherapy.* Boston: Houghton Mifflin.

Rogers, C. R. (1951) *Client-Centred Therapy.* London: Constable.

Rogers, C. R. (1961). *On Becoming a Person.* Boston: Houghton Mifflin.

Rosen, H. J., Perry, R. J., Murphy, J., Kramer, J. H., Mychack, P. et al (2002) Emotion comprehension in the temporal variant of frontotemporal dementia. *Brain*, 125(10), pp 2286–95.

Ruch, G. (2005) Relationship-based practice and reflective practice: holistic approaches to contemporary child care social work. *Child and Family Social Work*, 10, pp 111–23.

Rusting, C. L. (2001) Personality as a moderator of affective influences on cognition. In Forgas, J. P. (Ed.) *Affect and Social Cognition.* Mahwah, NJ: Lawrence Erlbaum Associates, pp 371–91.

Rutter, M. (1979) Protective factors in children's responses to stress and disadvantage. In M. W. Kent and J. E. Rolf (Eds.) *Primary Prevention in Psychopathology. Vol. 3: Social Competence in Children.* Hanover, NH: University Press of New England, pp 49–74.

Rutter, M. (1990) Psychosocial resilience and protective mechanisms. In J. Rolf, A. S. Masten, D. Cicchetti, K. H. Nuechterlin and S. Weintraub (Eds.) *Risk and Protective Factors in the Development of Psychopathology.* New York: Cambridge University Press, pp 181–214.

Rutter, M. (2006) *Genes and Behavior: Nature–Nurture Interplay Explained.* Oxford: Blackwell.

Saarni, C. (2000) Emotional competence: a developmental perspective. In R. Bar-On and J. D. A. Parker (Eds). *The Handbook of Emotional Intelligence*, San Francisco: Jossey Bass, pp 68–91.

Sainsbury, E. (1975) *Social Work with Families: Perceptions of Social Casework among Clients of a Family Service Unit.* Routledge and Kegan Paul: London.

Sainsbury, E., Nixon, S. and Phillips, D. (1982) *Social Work in Focus: Clients' and Social Workers' Perceptions of in Long Term Work.* London: Routledge and Kegan Paul.

Salovey, P., Brackett, M. A. and Mayer, J. D. (Eds.) (2004) *Emotional Intelligence: Key Readings on the Mayer and Salovey Model.* Port Chester, New York: Dude Publishing.

Salovey, P. and Mayer, J. (1990) Emotional intelligence. *Imagination, Cognition and Personality*, 9, pp 185–211.

Salovey, P. and Mayer, J. (2004) 'What is emotional intelligence?' In P. Salovey, M. A. Brackett and J. D. Mayer (Eds.) (2004) *Emotional Intelligence:*

Key Readings on the Mayer and Salovey Model. Dude Publishing: New York, pp 29–47.

Salzberger-Wittenberg, I. (1970) *Psycho-Analytic Insight and Relationships: A Kleinian Approach*. London: Routledge.

Sapolsky, R. M. (1998) *Why Zebras Don't Get Ulcers*. New York: W. H. Freeman.

Schore, A. (1994) *Affect Regulation and the Origins of the Self: The Neurobiology of Emotional Development*. Hillsdale, NJ.: Erlbaum.

Schore, A. (2001a) Effects of a secure attachment relationship on right brain development, affect regulation, and infant mental health. *Infant Mental Health Journal*,22 (1–2), pp 7–66.

Schore, A. (2001b) The effects of early relational trauma on right brain development, affect regulation, and infant mental health. *Infant Mental Health Journal*, 22(1–2), pp 201–69.

Seligman, M. (1975) *Helplessness: On Depression, Development, and Death*. San Francisco: W. H. Freeman.

Seligman, M. (2003) *Authentic Happiness*. London: Nicholas Brealey.

Selye, H. (1956) *The Stress of Life*. New York: McGraw Hill.

Shoda, Y., Mischel, W. and Peake, P. K. (1990) Predicting adolescent cognitive and self-regulatory competences from preschool delay of gratification. *Developmental Psychology*, 26(6), pp 978–86.

Shoenberg, P. (2007) *Psychosomatics: The Uses of Psychotherapy*. Houndmills: Palgrave Macmillan.

Shulman, L. (1999) *The Skills of Helping: Individuals and Groups*. Illinois: Peacock.

Siegel, D. (1999) *The Developing Mind: Toward a Neurobiology of Interpersonal Experience*. New York: The Guilford Press.

Siegel, D. (2003) An interpersonal neurobiology of psychotherapy: the developing mind and the resolution of trauma. In M. Solomon and D. Siegel (Eds.) *Healing Trauma: Attachment, Mind, Body, and Brain*. New York: W. W. Norton, pp 1–56.

Smith, M. (2005) *Surviving Fears in Health and Social Care*. London: Jessica Kingsley.

Spiegal, D., Bloom, J., Kraemer, H., and Gottleil, E. (1989) Effect of psychosocial treatment on survival of patients with metastatic breast cancer. *Lancet*, 2(8668), pp 888–91.

Spratt, T. and Callan, J. (2004) Parents' views on social work interventions in child welfare cases. *British Journal of Social Work*, 34, pp 199–224.

Stemmler, G. (2004) Physiological processes during emotion. In P. Philippott and R. S. Feldman (Eds.) *The Regulation of Emotion*. Mahweh, NJ: Lawrence Erlbaum Associates, pp 33–70.

Stern, D. N. (1977) *The First Relationship: Infant and Mother*. Cambridge, MA: Harvard University Press.

Stern, D. N. (2004) *The Present Moment in Psychotherapy and Everyday Life*. New York: W. W. Norton.

Sternberg, E. M. (2001) *The Balance Within: The Science Connecting Health and Emotions.* New York: W. H. Freeman,

Sternberg, R. J. (1985) *Beyond IQ: A Triarchic Theory of Human Intelligence.* New York: Cambridge University Press.

Strupp, H., Fox, R. and Lessler, K. (1969) *Patients View their Psychotherapy.* Johns Hopkins University Press: Baltimore, MD.

Sudbery, J. (2002) Key features of therapeutic social work: the use of relationship. *Journal of Social work Practice*, 16(2), pp 149–62.

Taylor, G. J. and Bagby, R. M. (2000) An Overview of the alexithymia construct. In R. Bar-On and J. D. A. Parker (Eds.) *The Handbook of Emotional Intelligence.* San Francisco: Jossey Bass, pp 40–67.

Taylor, G. J., Bagby, R. M. and Parker, J. D. A. (1997) *Disorders of affect regulation.* Cambridge: Cambridge University Press.

Thomas, D. (1937/1971) Dylan Thomas: The Poems. London: J. M. Dent & Sons.

Thompson, R. A. (1995) *Preventing Child Maltreatment through Social Support.* Thousand Oaks: Sage.

Thorndike, E. L. (1920) Intelligence and its use. *Harper's Magazine*, 140, 227–35.

Thorne, B. (1997) Person-centred counselling. In M. Davies (Ed.) *The Blackwell Companion to Social Work.* Oxford: Blackwell, pp 177–84.

Tolstoy, L. (1875/2003) *Anna Karenina.* London: Penguin.

Tomkins, S. S. (1962) *Affect, Imagery, Consciousness: Vol 2, The Negative Affects.* New York: Springer-Verlag.

Tooby, J. and Cosmides, L. (1990) The past explains the present: emotional adaptations and the structure of ancestral environments. *Ethology and Sociobiology*, 11, pp 375–424.

Trevarthen, C. and Aitkin, K. (2001) Infant intersubjectivity: research, theory and clinical application, *Journal of Child Psychology and Psychiatry*, 42(1), pp 3–48.

Trevithick, P. (2003) Effective relationship-based practice: a theoretical explanation. *Journal of Social Work Practice*, 17(2), pp 163–76.

Truax, C. B. and Carkhuff, R. B. (1967) *Towards Effective Counselling and Psychotherapy*, Aldine: Chicago.

van der Kolk, B. (2003) Post traumatic stress disorder and the nature of trauma. In M. Solomon and D. Siegel (Eds.) *Healing Trauma: Attachment, Mind, Body, and Brain.* New York: W. W. Norton, pp 168–95.

Wallerstein, J. (1986) Women after divorce: a preliminary report from a ten-year follow up. *American Journal of Orthopsychiatry*, 56, pp 65–77.

Watson, J. B. and Raynor, R. (1920) Condition emotional reactions. *Journal of Experimental Psychology*, 3, pp 1–14.

Webster-Stratton, C. (1999) *How to Promote Children's Social and Emotional Competence.* Thousand Oaks: Sage/Paul Chapman Publishing.

Wilkinson, R. (2000) *Mind the Gap: Hierarchies, Health and Human Evolution.* London: Weidenfeld and Nicolson.

Williams, N. L., Reardon, J. M., Murray, K. T. and Cole, T. M. (2005) Anxiety disorders: a developmental vulnerability-stress perspective. In B. L. Hankin and J. R. Z. Abela (Eds.) *Development of Psychopathology: A Vulnerability-Stress Perspective.* Thousand Oaks: Sage, pp 289–327.

Winnicott, D. (1960) The theory of the parent–infant relationship. In *The Maturational Process and the Facilitating Environment.* New York: International Universities Press, pp 37–55.

Winnicott, D. (1965) *The Maturational Process and the Facilitative Environment.* New York: International Universities Press.

Winnicott, D. (1967) Mirror-role of mother and family in child development. In P. Lomas (Ed.) *The Predicament of the Family.* London: Hogarth Press, pp 26–33.

Wolfe, D. A. (1999) *Child Abuse: Implications for Children, Development and Psychopathology* (2nd ed.). Thousand Oaks, CA, US: Sage Publications.

Wolpe, J. (1990) *The Practice of Behavior Therapy* (4th ed.). New York: Pergamon.

Wolpert, L. (1999) *Malignant Sadness: The Anatomy of Depression.* London: Faber and Faber.

Woodward, J. (1988) *Understanding Ourselves: The Uses of Therapy.* London: Macmillan Press.

Zech, E., Rimé, B. and Nils, F. (2004) Social sharing of emotion, emotional recovery, and interpersonal aspects. In P. Philippott and R. S. Feldman (Eds.) *The Regulation of Emotion.* Mahweh, NJ: Lawrence Erlbaum Associates, pp 157–85.

Zirkel, S. (2000) Social intelligence. In R. Bar-On and J. D. A. Parker (Eds.) *The Handbook of Emotional Intelligence.* San Francisco: Jossey Bass, pp 3–27.

Name Index

Subject Index